JENNY RUHL

Blood Sugar 101

What They Don't Tell You About Diabetes

Second Edition

TECHNION Books

Published by Technion Books
P.O. Box 402
Turners Falls, MA 01376
technionbooks@outlook.com

This publication is sold with the understanding that the publisher and author are not engaged in rendering medical or other professional services. **If medical advice or other expert assistance is required, the services of a competent professional person should be sought.**

ISBN-13: 978-0-9647116-6-2
ISBN-10: 0-9647116-6-4

Printed in the United States of America

Table of Contents

Preface to the Second Edition

Over the eight years that have passed since the first edition of this book was published, there have been significant changes in how doctors treat patients with Type 2 Diabetes. This has made it necessary to do a major revision of this text.

Most of these changes have occurred in response to the flood of new, expensive, patented drugs that have come to market over this period. In many cases they have replaced the drugs that were popular almost a decade ago when the first edition of this book was released.

Fortunately for the readers of the earlier edition, the scientific discoveries that have occurred during this period have only strengthened the case for the approach we took in the original version of this book. The simple, moderate, but powerful approach to diet we laid out still works brilliantly. Hardly a day passes when I don't hear from readers who write to tell me of the dramatic improvements they have made in their health after following the advice you will read in these pages. They have lowered their blood sugars to normal levels, lost weight, healed painful feet, and kept their eyes and kidneys healthy.

In addition, with the insights they have gained from these pages, these readers have learned how to evaluate any new strategy their doctors might recommend, be it taking a brand new drug, trying an innovative but extreme diet, or choosing an irreversible surgical intervention.

In this new edition, you will still find the information and advice they found so helpful, along with a greatly expanded discussion of the pros and cons of the many new drugs that have recently entered the marketplace. You will also learn more about what researchers have learned about currently fashionable dietary and surgical approaches your doctor might suggest to you. We have also added several new research-based insights that can help you make healthier choices when choosing from the many foods that will lower your blood sugar.

It is our hope that this new edition will give another generation of readers the tools they need to join the growing ranks of those who have overcome diabetes and restored themselves to completely normal health.

Introduction

Type 2 Diabetes is a terrible disease. It causes impotence, blindness, kidney failure, amputation, and heart attack death.

But Type 2 Diabetes is also a wonderful disease because all these dreadful outcomes are optional. No matter how severe your diabetes might be at diagnosis, it is unique among the serious chronic diseases in that it is the *only* condition where you, the patient, with only a small amount of help from your doctor and no heroic medical interventions can achieve normal health.

This is probably not what you have heard from your doctors. They probably told you it is *normal* for someone with diabetes to suffer foot pain, impotence, slow wound healing, low physical energy, and even a heart attack. So why should you believe me when I tell you it isn't true?

For a very good reason: Over the past two decades diabetes treatment has been revolutionized by the emergence of what is often called "The Wisdom of the Web." This term refers to the phenomenon where many thousands of people, each drawing on their own knowledge and experience, create information resources as good or better than those produced by so-called authorities.

Diabetes on the Web

Diabetes was one of the first diseases to benefit from the Wisdom of the Web because people with diabetes have always been expected to do most of the work involved in managing their disease. They've tested their own blood sugar. They've adjusted their own insulin doses. So even before the advent of the Web they had a lot of information about how their blood sugar responded to changes in their diet, medications, and exercise. What they didn't have was any idea of how their own experience might compare with that of others.

With the emergence of the Web, people with diabetes began to talk to each other on newsgroups and discussion forums. They exchanged information they'd gotten from their solitary testing. They started comparing notes. When they did this, they soon discovered that they weren't the only ones who were having problems with the diets and drug regimens prescribed by doctors and dietitians.

Some people who were active on the Web started trying out alternative diets and drug regimens and reporting their results to each other in the discussion groups. Others started combing through the thousands of peer-reviewed journal articles that had been made available for free on the Web, searching for studies that might point to more effective diabetes treatments. Over time, using the information they found and shared made big improvements in their health.

The 5% Club

Since my own diabetes diagnosis in 1998 I have participated in thousands of Web discussions with hundreds of people with diabetes. Like myself, many of them had science, software, or engineering backgrounds. This gave them a penchant for critical thinking and the skills needed to read and understand journal research. Working together, we learned that it *is* possible for people with diabetes to achieve normal blood sugars. We also uncovered research that suggests that if we maintain truly normal blood sugars we will avoid or even reverse the terrible complications our doctors told us were inevitable.

Some of us call ourselves "The 5% Club" because our goal was to keep our A1c test results under 6%. That is the level most doctors consider to be the normal range. Using a selection of techniques I've learned from participating in Web discussion groups, I've managed to stay in The 5% Club for almost all of the 18 years that have followed my diagnosis. Though it has been that long since I was diagnosed, my endocrinologist sometimes refers to me as "recently diagnosed" because she is used to seeing A1cs that low only in people who are new to diabetes.

Why This Book?

In 2005, after realizing that many people were unaware of the wealth of information to be found in Web discussion groups, I decided to put the most important information on a Web site where people doing Google searches could easily find it. The heart of my Web site was what I'd learned after spending several months reading through medical journals, hunting for studies that answered two questions: "What is a truly normal blood sugar level?" and "What blood sugar levels cause organ damage?" The result was my web site **Bloodsugar101.com**.

This site is different from most other diabetes web sites because the information you find on it includes links to studies published in top-rated peer-reviewed medical journals. Visitors to the site don't have to take anything on trust. They can follow the links and read the research papers themselves. My web site is also updated any time something significant turns up in the medical news that is relevant to a topic discussed on its pages.

Over the years, the site grew huge. Visitors started asking me if I could put the mass of information stored on the web site into book form so they could read it more easily. They explained that because the site has grown so large, they could not read the whole thing on the web and worried that they might be missing out on critical pieces of information buried in its pages.

Since I had already published seven previous books of nonfiction, including a business bestseller, I was excited by the challenge of turning the site into a book. My enthusiasm for the project grew when I began to write it, as I began to see another advantage to putting what I'd written about diabetes into book form: A book is better than a web site at explaining ideas that can't be compressed into a few simple paragraphs, because the sequential structure of a book ensures that every concept you encounter in its pages builds on what you have already read. A book is also free of the distractions inherent in the web's hypertextual design.

Since its original launch in 2008, it has become clear that this book adds value to the web site by providing, in a compact and portable form, an orderly examination of the crucial concepts that pervade it. In its pages you will find the explanations that will make you understand, as you never have before, how your blood sugar works, what happens when your blood sugar control breaks down, what blood sugar levels damage your organs, and how you can safely lower your blood sugar enough to prevent any further diabetic complications from occurring.

Every scientific concept presented in the text is backed up by peer-reviewed research papers that were published in highly regarded medical journals. If you want check out this research, you can find the citations in the "References" section at the end of this book. You can find the links to these studies and to any new relevant scientific findings online at **Bloodsugar101.com**. You can also keep up with important new research published since this book went to press by following the blog, "Updates to Blood Sugar 101." That blog can be found at: **http://phlauntdiabetesupdates.blogspot.com**

However, there are some very important issues that people with diabetes must deal with that are not discussed in peer-reviewed research. Here the Wisdom of the Web comes into play as I draw on the experiences reported by the hundreds of knowledgeable people with diabetes who have posted messages on the web over the decades. When I cite this type of information, I make it clear that anecdotal reports are its source.

No One Way

Unlike most other diabetes books on the market, this book does not tell you what to eat or what medications to take. If there is one thing we have learned from the Wisdom of the web, it is that each of us is different and that a strategy that works well for one person may not work for another.

Instead we will teach you how to tell if *any* diabetes strategy you are using is working. By "working" we mean giving you blood sugars low enough to prevent any further organ damage. We'll show you how to find out if your current diabetes diet is doing the job and, if it isn't, we'll show you how to improve it. If you need more than a change of diet to get your blood sugars back into the safe zone, we'll explore what the diabetes drugs available to you are good for and discuss their drawbacks, putting particular emphasis on some cheap but effective diabetes drugs that doctors may overlook because they aren't being promoted by drug company marketing campaigns.

What's in It for You?

When you are done reading this book, you will know enough to hold an intelligent conversation with your doctor about your treatment choices. You'll be better able to evaluate the latest "breakthroughs" you read about in the diabetes news. And most importantly, you'll have the information you need to keep yourself safe, no matter what current fad is sweeping the medical community. In short, when you are done with this book, you will have the tools you need to join "The 5% Club." So welcome aboard!

Chapter One
What is Normal Blood Sugar?

Diabetes is not a disease, it's a symptom.

Everyone diagnosed with any type of diabetes shares a single symptom with every other person with diabetes. That symptom is high blood sugar.

Anything that interferes with the complex mechanisms that the body uses to regulate blood sugar may cause diabetes. It may occur when the cells that secrete insulin get poisoned and die off or when those cells fail to respond to the signals that tell them to make insulin. It may even occur when those cells are making plenty of insulin but insulin receptors in the cells have lost their ability to respond to it. Diabetes can be caused by abnormalities of the adrenal glands or problems with hormones in the gut that inform the body of the presence of food.

It is also possible for one person to have more than one of these metabolic problems at the same time. For example, the most common form of diabetes, which doctors call Type 2 Diabetes, is frequently described as being caused by insulin resistance, the condition where cell receptors stop responding properly to insulin. But scientists have recently discovered that almost one in twelve of those diagnosed with insulin resistant Type 2 Diabetes also have markers in their bloodstream that show they have been the victim of an autoimmune attack that has killed off the cells that make insulin.

What does this mean for you?

Simply this: Though you may have been diagnosed with diabetes, all that your diabetes, my diabetes, and the diabetes of the person sitting across from you at the diabetes support group meeting have in common is that they cause all of us to have abnormally high blood sugars. The causes of our high blood sugars may be different, how high our blood sugars rise after we eat the identical meal may be different, how our bodies respond to the same dose of the same drug may be dramatically different, and, most importantly, what it takes to bring our blood sugars back into the normal range, which prevents complications, will be different.

Because we are all so different, the key to recovering good health is to figure out how your own individual version of diabetes works. The first step toward doing this is to learn how blood sugar is regulated in a normal person and how normal blood sugar control breaks down. Armed with this information you will be better able to understand what the various interventions used to treat diabetes do—and which ones might be right for you. So take the time to understand the information you'll find in the next couple pages. It will give you the background you need to take control of your health.

Blood Sugar Control in Normal People

All your cells require a steady supply of fuel to continue functioning. The most essential of these fuels is a sugar called glucose. It is the sugar we refer to as **blood sugar**. Some glucose always circulates in the bloodstream, where it is available to any cell that might need it. Though most cells can survive by burning fat when no glucose is available, important cells in your brain cannot. Deprived of a steady supply of glucose for as little as five minutes these cells will die and so will you. So keeping a steady supply of glucose flowing in your veins is essential to survival.

When you read that your blood sugar is 100 mg/dl, what this is really telling you is that there are 100 milligrams of glucose—one tenth of a gram—in every deciliter of your blood. A deciliter is one tenth of a liter. So if your blood sugar is 100 mg/dl you have 1 gram of glucose in every liter of blood.

Everywhere except in the United States, the concentration of glucose in your blood is measured using a different unit: mmol/L, which stands for millimoles per liter. To convert mg/dl into mmol/L you divide mg/dl by 18.05. Appendix A gives you a table you can use to find the mmol/L equivalent of any blood sugar mentioned in these pages.

Before most cells can use glucose, it must be transported inside the cells. Insulin is the hormone that makes this happen. That is why insulin is so important to blood sugar control. If there is no insulin available, no matter how much glucose is circulating in your bloodstream most of your cells will not be able to use it. And if the sugar in your blood isn't taken into cells, it will build up to dangerously high levels that will damage your organs and can even lead to death.

Insulin is produced by special cells called **beta cells**. These tiny cells are found in structures called the Islets of Langerhans, which are scattered throughout your pancreas. The pancreas is an organ located near your liver that also secretes digestive enzymes. The job of the beta cell is to manufacture insulin, store it, and release it into the bloodstream when appropriate. Healthy beta cells are continually making insulin and storing it within the beta cell in the form of tiny granules.

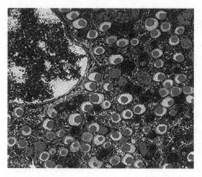

The beta cells release this insulin into the bloodstream in two different ways. They release a continuous trickle of what is called **Basal Insulin** throughout the day and they also release larger bursts of insulin after you eat a meal. The meal time releases are called **First- and Second-Phase Insulin Release**.

Basal Insulin Release

Figure 1. Beta cells in an Islet of Langerhans. The beta cells in this picture are marked with gray dots

The purpose of basal insulin release is to keep a small amount of insulin flowing in the bloodstream at all times. The beta cells of a healthy person release insulin into the bloodstream in small pulses that occur every few minutes throughout the day and night. Scientists have discovered that even when beta cells are capable of producing insulin, diabetes may develop when something disrupts the timing of this pulsed basal insulin release.

During periods between meals healthy beta cells also manufacture extra insulin and store it in the form of granules for use at meal time. Problems with basal insulin production can also keep the beta cells from storing these granules of insulin. This will make it much harder to avoid high blood sugar peaks after meals.

When you test your **fasting blood sugar** after not eating for eight hours or more, you are checking your ability to secrete basal insulin. A normal or near normal fasting blood sugar means that your ability to secrete basal insulin is still intact. Truly normal fasting blood sugar values fall in the range between 70 and 85 mg/dl. Doctors will tell you that the normal range for a fasting blood sugar extends up to 100 mg/dl, but research has shown that people whose fasting blood sugar is over 92 mg/dl are much more likely to develop diabetes within a decade, which suggests that it is not truly normal.

Insulin Levels Signal the Liver Whether More Glucose Is Needed

One of the liver's important functions is to top off the level of glucose in the blood if it starts to drop too low. When basal insulin production is working properly, the steady flow of insulin it supplies to the bloodstream sends the signal to the liver that all is well and that no more glucose is needed. But if the insulin level drops during a fasting period, or if the liver becomes insulin resistant and does not respond to insulin signaling, the liver will assume that the glucose in the bloodstream is almost used up and more glucose is needed.

To supply that glucose, the liver turns to **glycogen**, a starchy carbohydrate that it has stored for just this purpose. **Carbohydrates** are a group of edible molecules that include sugars, starches, and some kinds of fiber. Glycogen is made up of a long chain of glucose molecules that have been bonded together. When the liver needs to raise the blood sugar, it converts this glycogen back into glucose and then dumps that glucose into the bloodstream. This raises the blood sugar back to its normal level and ensures that cells will continue to have the fuel they need.

If the liver doesn't have enough glycogen stored, it can convert protein into glucose, too. First it will convert protein derived from food you have recently eaten. If you aren't eating enough protein, the body will break down the protein that makes up your muscles to get the glucose you need. This ability of the liver to turn muscle into glucose is why dieters on stringent diets lose muscle mass if they don't eat enough protein.

First-Phase Insulin Release

As soon as a healthy person starts to eat a meal, the parasympathetic nervous system sends out signals that begin the process that causes beta cells to release insulin into the bloodstream, beginning with the insulin they previously stored in granules.

As food reaches the stomach, the carbohydrates in that food start to digest. Any pure glucose that's been eaten goes immediately into the blood stream, as it doesn't need to be broken down any further. Pure fructose gets whisked away to the liver, which converts it into fat. Digestive enzymes then break down the rest of the complex sugars and starches supplied by the meal into the two simple sugars, glucose and fructose. That glucose goes into the bloodstream, too. It takes no more than 15 minutes after a person has eaten a meal containing sugar or starch for the first glucose from the digested food to reach their bloodstream and begin raising the concentration of glucose in their blood.

Rising blood sugars now stimulate the beta cells to secrete more insulin. At the same time, as blood sugars rise to a threshold—somewhere between 100 and 120 mg/dl—**incretin hormones** released by the gut also stimulate the beta cells to secrete insulin. These early releases of insulin that occur as soon as we begin eating a meal are called **first-phase insulin release**. In a healthy person first-phase insulin release keeps the blood sugar from rising much over 125 mg/dl.

What cells take up that glucose? The brain and muscles have first dibs. Then the liver will use some glucose to top off its store of glycogen. But if your brain and muscle cells have enough glucose, and your liver has enough glycogen, insulin pushes glucose into *fat* cells. Insulin plays an important part in the process that transforms glucose into fat.

The amount of insulin a normal person's beta cells secrete during this first-phase insulin release is believed to be very close to the amount they needed to process the glucose produced by previous meals. If they usually eat a lot of carbohydrate, their body will release more insulin at the start of the next meal, even if that meal doesn't contain much carbohydrate. If this large dose of first-phase insulin doesn't meet up with enough incoming carbohydrate, it may drive the normal person's blood sugar low. When blood sugar drops too low, the brain senses it and sends out hunger signals that ramp up carbohydrate cravings. This is suggested as a reason why people with normal or near-normal metabolisms who have been eating a lot of carbohydrate may find themselves craving carbohydrates if they try to cut down on their carbohydrate intake.

If the normal person doesn't respond to the low blood sugar attack by eating more carbohydrate, their liver will transform more stored glycogen into glucose and release that glucose into the blood stream until it has raised the blood sugar back to a normal level. When that person eats the next meal after the meal that resulted in a low blood sugar, their beta cells will release less first-phase insulin and avoid causing another low blood sugar.

In a healthy person, the first-phase insulin release peaks shortly after they've started their meal. The highest blood sugar level they will experience usually occurs by 45 minutes after they started eating.

The rising insulin level in the blood caused by this first-phase insulin release also signals the liver that there is no need to add additional glucose to the blood, shutting down the glucose dumping the liver does during periods of fasting.

Second-Phase Insulin Release

After completing this first-phase insulin release, the beta cells pause. But if the blood sugar is still not back under 100 mg/dl ten to twenty minutes later, beta cells start to secrete more insulin and provide another, smaller, **second-phase insulin release** whose job is to mop up the rest of the excess glucose circulating in the bloodstream. This second-phase insulin release continues as long as it is needed—until the blood sugar is back down to its fasting level. In a normal person, this usually takes about an hour to an hour and a half after the start of a meal.

It is this combination of a robust first-phase insulin release of stored insulin and a strong second-phase insulin release of secreted insulin that keeps the blood sugar of a normal person almost always under 100 mg/dl except for the first hour following a meal. This system ensures that the brain and organs get a steady supply of glucose to fill their needs but prevents the build up of excess glucose in the blood stream that might clog up capillaries, gum up the kidneys, or inhibit the activity of nerves.

What Are Truly Normal Blood Sugar Levels?

An illuminating research study presented by Professor J. S. Christiansen at the European Association for the Study of Diabetes conference in September of 2006 depicted the daily pattern of blood sugars in a group of normal subjects as it was revealed by the use of a **Continuous Glucose Monitoring System** (CGMS). The CGMS is a small computer attached to a probe. The probe is inserted under the skin where it samples the blood sugar every few minutes for a period lasting from a few days to several weeks. The computer stores and graphs this information.

Dr. Christiansen's data is summarized in Figure 2. A group of normal people wore the CGMS during the period spanning from when they woke up and ate breakfast until just before lunch. The heavy line shows the median blood sugar of the group as a whole. Next to it are thinner lines showing the top and bottom of the range within which most of their blood sugars fell. The lower set of lines represents their insulin and C-peptide levels. (C-peptide is a byproduct of the manufacture of insulin. Measuring it is a way of measuring insulin production.) The vertical line indicates the time when the study subjects ate a high carbohydrate breakfast.

The data collected from these normal people shows how throughout the night their median fasting blood glucose concentration remained flat in the low 80 mg/dl range. After a high carbohydrate meal, their blood sugar rose to a median value near 125 mg/dl for a brief period. This occurred about 45 minutes after they ate. In all but the people with the highest readings, blood sugar dropped back under 100 mg/dl by one hour and fifteen minutes after eating and it returned to 85 mg/dl by one hour and forty-five minutes after eating.

Note that even the highest of these normal readings is far below the cutoff most doctors consider to be the high end of "normal." That cutoff, established decades before continuous glucose monitoring was available and based on outdated data, is still officially defined as being 139 mg/dl measured *two hours after eating*!

Figure 2. CGMS Study: Normal Blood Sugars

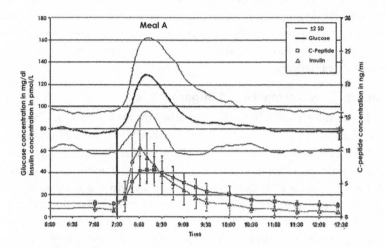

Chapter Two
How Diabetes Develops

Now that you understand how the normal body controls blood sugar levels, it's time to look at what happens when that control breaks down. Before we do that, we need to take a moment to discuss the tests doctors and researchers use to measure blood sugar performance and to learn the terms doctors use to describe the various stages of deterioration that lie between normalcy and diabetes, so we can better understand the research that explores this issue.

The Blood Sugar Tests Doctors Use

Table 1 shows the diagnostic criteria used to distinguish between normal blood sugar, prediabetes, and full-fledged diabetes. The fasting criteria have changed several times, so current and historical ranges are both given. These criteria are set and periodically updated by a committee of experts appointed by the American Diabetes Association. All values are given in mg/dl.

Test	Normal	Prediabetes	Diabetes
Fasting Plasma Glucose (Current)	70-99	100 - 125	126+
Fasting Plasma Glucose (Before 1998)	70-110	110 – 139	140+
2-Hr OGTT (1978 – Today)	70 -139	140-199	200+

Table 1. Ranges for Diagnosing Blood Sugar Disorders, in mg/dl

Fasting Plasma Glucose

Though, as we have seen above, continuous glucose monitors give a very clear picture of exactly how blood sugar behaves throughout the day, they are expensive and complicated to use, so researchers and doctors rarely use them when evaluating patients' blood sugar. Instead they use a few standardized tests that are far less precise. One is the **fasting plasma glucose** test, abbreviated **FPG**. This is a simple test that requires only a single blood draw. It measures the concentration of glucose in the blood after an eight hour fast. The FPG only gives information about how the blood sugar behaves in the *fasting* state.

The American Diabetes Association has defined some arbitrary values to be applied when using this test to determine if a person's blood sugar is normal, if they have an intermediate form of blood sugar dysfunction called **impaired fasting glucose (IFG)**, or if they have diabetes.

The ADA's definition of what fasting plasma glucose test values should be used for making these diagnoses has changed over the years. Until 1998 the ADA defined a fasting plasma glucose of 140 mg/dl or more as being diabetic. In 1998 they lowered the diabetes diagnostic cutoff to 126 mg/dl. The ADA has also lowered the value used to define the upward limit of normal several times. Its current value is 99 mg/dl.

This is why studies conducted before 1998 did not consider people to be diabetic unless their fasting blood sugars were over 140 mg/dl. Now that the diagnostic cutoff for the fasting plasma glucose test has dropped to 126 mg/dl, we know that a lot of people considered nondiabetic in older studies were actually diabetic, so some caution needs to be used when interpreting older studies.

The Oral Glucose Tolerance Test

The test used to track how first- and second-phase insulin releases are holding up is the **Oral Glucose Tolerance Test (OGTT)**. It measures how a person's blood sugar responds after they consume a huge dose of pure glucose. Unlike food, glucose doesn't need to be digested and goes directly into the bloodstream. Because of this, the blood sugar patterns seen during an OGTT can be very different from those you see when testing your blood sugar after meals. The OGTT may cause intense blood sugar peaks that can be more severe than those you experience when eating the same amount of carbohydrate in the form of real food. But these peaks may resolve far more quickly, too. Reactive lows are also more common after an OGTT than when eating carbohydrate-rich foods that digest more slowly.

The procedure for administering an OGTT is this: Subjects who have been fasting are given a fasting plasma glucose test. They then drink a glass containing 75 grams of glucose dissolved in water. After this, their blood sugar is measured at set intervals, usually one hour and two hours after drinking the glucose. However, to save money, many doctors only order the two hour measurement.

If a person's blood sugar is 140 mg/dl or higher two hours after drinking the glucose, the person is considered to have **prediabetes** or **impaired glucose tolerance (IGT)**. People whose blood sugar is under

140 mg/dl at two hours are considered to be normal, though there is no functional difference between what is happening in the body of the "normal" person whose blood sugar is 139 mg/dl two hours after drinking glucose and in that of the "prediabetic" person whose blood sugar at two hours is 140 mg/dl.

During the OGTT, if the blood sugar reading is higher than 199 mg/dl at two hours, the person is diagnosed as diabetic. Again, this is not because there is any functional difference between a blood sugar that rises to 199 mg/dl and one that goes to 200 mg/dl, but simply because the ADA's Expert Panel arbitrarily chose this number as the level at which they would diagnose diabetes.

In discussing medical studies, if a single OGTT result is cited it should be assumed to be a two hour test result unless it is specifically described otherwise.

The A1c Test

The test your doctor is most likely to rely on to track your blood sugar control is the **A1c** test, also called the **Hemoglobin A₁c** test and abbreviated hgA₁c. Both the test and its result are often just referred to as "the A1c." The A1c is a cheap test that can be administered—and billed—by your doctor's office. It is frequently used to measure blood sugar control in studies of large populations where it would be too expensive to perform individual glucose tolerance tests.

The A1c doesn't measure the concentration of sugar in your blood. Instead, it measures something else: how much glucose has become permanently bonded to the hemoglobin in your red blood cells. For most, but not all, people this will reflect how their high blood sugar has been, on average, during the past couple months. The reason that the amount of glucose bonded to your red blood cells can provide a measurement of your blood sugar levels over time is because the higher your blood sugar has been over an extended period, the more likely it is that glucose carried in your bloodstream will become permanently bonded to your hemoglobin. The A1c test result is expressed as a percentage, since it reflects the percentage of red blood cells that have glucose permanently bonded to them.

A normal A1c falls between 4.0 and 5.0%. People with diabetes usually have A1cs ranging from 6.0% to as high as 15.0%.

Doctors use various formulas to estimate the average blood sugar they believe matches your A1c test result. The formula believed to be the most accurate is the ADAG formula, which was derived from CGMS studies. It is:

$$\text{Average Glucose in mg/dl} = (28.7 \times \text{A1c}) - 46.7$$

Because red blood cells usually live around 3 months, most doctors believe that the A1c reflects three months' worth of blood sugar control. However, studies suggest the A1c largely reflects your blood sugar control over the two weeks before you took the test. Studies have also found that in people with near normal blood sugars the height of post-meal blood sugar spikes greatly influences the A1c result. Only in people whose A1cs approach 7.0% does the fasting blood sugar play a larger part in raising the A1c.

The A1c test will only reflect your average blood sugar control if you have a normal population of red blood cells. If you are anemic, by definition you have an abnormally low number of hemoglobin cells. This means you'll also have a deceptively low A1c reading no matter how high your blood sugars have been in the period before the test.

A1c test results are also likely to be misleading in people of non-white ethnicity who register higher A1cs at the same blood sugar levels.

Your A1c result may also be inaccurate if your red blood cells live longer or shorter than usual. Long-lived red blood cells can give a falsely high A1c reading because they continue to collect glucose during their longer lives. If your red blood cells are living shorter lives, they have less time to collect glucose. People with certain genetic variants of the red blood cell, including those with the sickle cell trait or Thalassemia, also will get misleadingly low A1c results. It is also possible that red blood cells live longer in people who keep their blood sugar under control, which may explain why some people who control their blood sugar tightly always see higher A1cs than are predicted by their blood sugar meter readings.

If your A1c test result predicts blood sugar levels dramatically different from what you see when you test your blood sugar at home with a meter, your doctor should order the **fructosamine** test instead of the A1c test. It is accurate in people with abnormal red blood cells.

If your doctor measures your A1c in the office, the result may also be misleading, because research has found that most of the instant A1c test kits marketed to doctors are much less accurate than lab tests. When in doubt, ask to have your A1c tested at a lab.

The Patterns in Which Diabetes Develops

Now it's time to learn how normal blood sugar deteriorates into diabetes. We'll start out by looking at what two long-lasting studies of large populations have taught us about the stages in which blood sugar control breaks down. Then we'll examine what is actually happening in your body during each of these stages.

A Landmark Study of Middle Aged People

Data from the Baltimore Longitudinal Study of Aging shows that over a period of ten years, the blood sugars of 48% of a large group of people in their 50s remained normal. Of the rest, 52% developed abnormal blood sugars, including the 11% who developed blood sugars high enough to be diagnosed as diabetic.

Outcome for 437 Originally Normal Subjects over a Decade of Observation Baltimore Longitudinal Study of Aging				
Normal	IGT only	IGT and IFG	IFG only	Diabetes
48%	31%	3%	5%	11%

Table 2. Percentage of Middle Aged Subjects Developing Impaired Fasting Glucose (IFG), Impaired Glucose Tolerance (IGT), and Diabetes.

By far the most prevalent pattern of blood sugar deterioration found in this group was the development of *impaired glucose tolerance with normal fasting blood sugar*. (The upper cutoff for normal fasting blood sugar used in this study was 110 mg/dl.) People with this pattern had blood sugars higher than 140 mg/dl when given a two hour OGTT, but their fasting blood sugars remained under 110 mg/dl. This suggests they were also very likely to also have blood sugars well over 140 mg/dl two hours after eating any meal containing a lot of carbohydrate.

Only 5% of the study subjects—one in twenty, developed the reverse pattern: impaired *fasting* glucose occurring with normal glucose tolerance. Only 3% simultaneously developed both impaired glucose tolerance and impaired fasting glucose. This makes it clear that it is far more common for *post-meal* blood sugar response to deteriorate before *fasting* blood sugar becomes impaired.

The Most Common Pattern for Those Developing Type 2 Diabetes

When the researchers turned their attention to the subset of people with abnormal blood sugars who had gone on to develop full-fledged diabetes, they found that, like the group as a whole, they were much more likely to get abnormal two hour glucose tolerance test results while still having normal Fasting Plasma Glucoses. Only a small number developed impaired fasting glucose while maintaining normal glucose tolerance.

This makes it very clear that deterioration of glucose tolerance — which implies deterioration in how blood sugar rises after a meal — is often the only apparent sign that a person is heading toward diabetes. For most people, the fasting blood sugar stays normal long after the meal-time control has faded out.

Of critical importance, in this study, *two thirds* of the people who were diagnosed as having diabetes using the glucose tolerance test had not yet developed impaired fasting glucose. Unfortunately, most doctors use *only* the fasting blood sugar test to screen patients for diabetes since it is cheap and very easy to administer, unlike the time-consuming OGTT. This is why doctors often don't diagnose people with diabetes until they've experienced years of deterioration.

So if you or a loved one are at risk for having diabetes you must insist that your doctor test your post-meal blood sugar, either with a blood sugar meter in the office or with an OGTT. If that isn't possible, buy a blood sugar meter yourself and test your blood sugar at home after meals. That way you can learn if you have abnormal post-meal blood sugars early on, when you can still intervene, preserve your fasting blood sugar control, and avoid developing early diabetic complications.

The Risk of Diabetes

The Baltimore Longitudinal Study of Aging diabetes study also found that a person in their fifties who has normal blood sugar has roughly a 1 in 8 chance of becoming diabetic over the next decade. A person who already has impaired glucose tolerance has a 4 in 10 chance of progressing to diabetes over a decade, while a person with impaired fasting glucose has almost a 1 in 2 chance of progressing to diabetes. Again, this suggests that fasting blood sugar control is the last part of blood sugar control to deteriorate.

Who Progresses?

The Baltimore Longitudinal Study of Aging data gives us some further insight into who develops diabetes in which pattern.

When analyzing data about the people who progressed to full-fledged diabetes, the researchers found that people older than 56 years were more likely to first develop impaired glucose tolerance than were younger people. The risk of developing impaired fasting glucose was about the same for all age groups.

They also found that men were more likely to see a deterioration in their fasting glucose than women, as were subjects with overall or central obesity when compared with lean subjects.

A Second Study Finds Diabetes Does Not Develop Gradually

A different study conducted in a large population looked at how the blood sugar of the *individuals* in that study changed over time.

The researchers studied a population of people living in Mexico City who were deemed to be at risk for diabetes. Every three years they measured the subjects' fasting plasma glucose and their fasting insulin levels. They also administered oral glucose tolerance tests.

A Swift and Unexpected Deterioration in Blood Sugar Control Precedes the Diagnosis of Diabetes

The researchers in this second study found that rather than being a gradual process, the transition to diabetes appeared to occur very quickly within a single three year period. One in twelve of the study subjects went from having normal glucose tolerance to having full-fledged diabetes during the three years between one examination and the next. Slightly fewer — one in fourteen — went from having impaired glucose tolerance to diabetes over the same three year period.

While the fasting plasma glucose of those who did *not* become diabetic increased "slightly and in an apparently linear manner," that of the people who became diabetic took a sudden step up, showing an average gain of 50 mg/dl between one examination and the next, three years later. The two hour oral glucose tolerance test results showed a similar pattern. The people who did *not* become diabetic showed a "slight increase" in their blood sugar values on the OGTT over the three year period, while those who became diabetic saw an average surge of 108 mg/dl between one exam and the next, three years later.

That this change was very sudden was highlighted by the discovery that the people who became diabetic during one three year period had shown very little change in their blood sugars over the three year period *before* the one in which their blood sugar deteriorated so swiftly. In fact, the changes in their blood sugar in that earlier period were the same as those in people who stayed normal.

This sudden loss of control probably occurs when first-phase insulin release fails. Research has shown that it is much harder to lower blood sugar when the rapid release of first-phase insulin is absent, because without the insulin signal, the liver continues to dump glucose during the meal.

What this study didn't discover, but many of us active on the web have found to be true, is that just as blood sugar control appears to deteriorate dramatically when you hit a certain high blood sugar threshold, when you take the steps needed to bring your post-meal blood sugars down below that critical level, you will often see a similarly dramatic rate of improvement.

What Happens at Each Stage of Breakdown?

Prediabetes/Impaired Glucose Tolerance

Remember the two stages of post-meal insulin release we described in Chapter One: The first-phase release of insulin that was previously stored in granules and the second-phase release of insulin secreted in real-time by your beta cells? Well, for most people, the first stage in the breakdown of blood sugar control happens when the first-phase insulin release after a meal stops working properly.

When you don't get a swift release of stored insulin as soon as you start to eat a meal containing carbohydrates, your blood sugar will rise much higher than a normal 125 mg/dl. Now all you can rely on to lower your post-meal blood sugar is the slower, weaker second-phase insulin release that only kicks in about a half hour after you start eating. This second-phase insulin release is slow because it requires your beta cells to secrete insulin rather than use the insulin they previously stored. Now, rather than peaking no more than 45 minutes after eating, the highest blood sugar you see after a meal will occur at least an hour after eating, possibly later. After it peaks, it may take another hour or longer for your blood sugar to return to normal.

This is clearly no longer normal. But it is not until the blood sugar remains above 139 mg/dl two hours after eating that doctors will diagnose **prediabetes**. A diagnosis of prediabetes is a very strong sign that your first-phase insulin release has been failing for a while and that you are now relying on second-phase insulin release to return your post-meal blood sugars to a normal level.

Many people remain prediabetic for the rest of their lives and never progress to diabetes. Even so, some may develop what doctors consider to be diabetic complications. This is because when you rely on your second-phase insulin release to control your blood sugar level after eating, it may take as many as three to five hours for your blood sugar level to return to normal. Since you eat every couple hours during the day, you will rarely get back to a truly normal blood sugar level between meals.

This is a huge problem, because, as you will see in Chapter Four, scientists have learned that hours of exposure to blood sugars in the so-called *prediabetic* range can cause *diabetic* complications.

Isolated Impaired Fasting Glucose

As was mentioned above, there is a small subset of people, mainly middle aged males, whose fasting glucose deteriorates first while their post-meal control remains normal. The reasons for this are not well understood, as little research has been done on isolated impaired fasting glucose. Some research has found that first-phase insulin secretion is impaired in these people too, though this is masked by the survival of a strong second-phase insulin release. Some of these may reach diabetic fasting blood sugar levels—over 125 mg/dl—while still having normal post-meal readings. Eventually, for many, this strong second-phase response fails, too, resulting in a swift passage from normal glucose tolerance to a fully diabetic post-meal response.

Others with isolated impaired fasting plasma glucose, however, may have a defect in a specific gene that only regulates fasting blood sugar levels. Unless they have other defective genes that affect blood sugar control, they are more likely to see their post-meal readings remain normal despite their elevated fasting values.

Impaired Fasting Glucose with Impaired Glucose Tolerance

More common is the pattern where impaired fasting glucose occurs along with impaired glucose tolerance. There's some evidence that for most of us it is the strain of coping with the loss of the first-phase insulin release that raises our fasting blood sugar. This is because when your post-meal blood sugars reach the diabetic range and your second-phase insulin release grows weaker, it may take four or five hours for your beta cells to secrete enough insulin to bring your blood sugar level down to its fasting level.

In fact, during the day, your blood sugar may never get back to a normal fasting level because glucose coming in from your next meal enters the bloodstream before glucose from the previous meal has been completely cleared. Only at night, while you are sleeping, will your beta cells finally be able to secrete enough insulin to lower your blood sugar enough to give you a normal fasting blood sugar.

However, since it took all the insulin your beta cells could make to lower you blood sugar to a normal level, your beta cells have had no chance to store any extra insulin to take care of your breakfast. As soon as you eat a bowl of cereal, your blood glucose will start to rise again. With no stored insulin to draw on, your beta cells will once again have to spend many hours secreting insulin to lower your blood sugar.

Eventually, even the long hours of the night will not provide enough time for your beta cells to produce the insulin you need to bring your blood sugar back to normal. Only then, perhaps a decade after you developed diabetic *post-meal* blood sugar readings, will you finally start seeing diabetic *fasting* blood sugar levels.

This process explains why, for most people who become diabetic, the fasting blood sugar level is the very last measurement to become abnormal. Only when your beta cells can't bring your blood sugar down to near-normal levels after eight long hours will you be diagnosed as diabetic by a doctor who relies on the fasting blood sugar test. This may mean that without knowing it you have been living with destructive, diabetic post-meal blood sugars for up to a decade before your doctor gives you a formal diagnosis.

Diabetes

The American Diabetes Association defines several different criteria for diagnosing diabetes. The most common is a reading over 200 mg/dl at two hours after the start of the OGTT. However, the ADA diagnostic criteria also state that a person should be diagnosed with diabetes when several random blood tests reveal a blood sugar level higher than 200 mg/dl at any time. Since many people whose sugars are spiking above 200 mg/dl after every meal have just enough second-phase insulin release to bring those levels down below 200 mg/dl two hours after eating, the random tests are a better diagnostic tool. Unfortunately, many doctors are unaware of that second criterion and will say you aren't diabetic even when your blood sugars are above 200 for several hours each day.

It is a mistake to wait until blood sugar remains above 200 mg/dl for more than two hours before beginning aggressive treatment for diabetes. Blood sugars that high are toxic to your remaining beta cells and will gradually kill them off. When that happens you will experience a dramatic surge to fasting readings above 200 mg/dl and post-meal levels of 300 mg/dl and more. Blood sugars at these levels are much harder to control, though they are common among people whose diabetes diagnoses have been delayed.

Why Blood Sugars Rise

Insulin Resistance

First- and second-phase insulin releases may fail to do their jobs for several reasons. The most common is the condition called **insulin resistance** in which receptors in the liver and the muscle cells stop responding properly to insulin. If high blood sugars are due solely to insulin resistance there may be a lot of insulin circulating in the body, but insulin resistant muscles or an insulin resistant liver don't respond to that insulin until its level rises abnormally high.

When a person's cells become insulin resistant, it takes a lot more insulin than normal to push circulating glucose into cells. In this case, while a person might have a perfectly normal first- and second-phase insulin release, the first-phase release might not produce enough insulin to clear all the circulating blood glucose that is produced after digesting a high carbohydrate meal.

The second-phase release might also be prolonged in an insulin resistant person because it takes a long time for beta cells to secrete the large amount of insulin needed to counter their insulin resistance. Eventually their body may not be able to produce enough insulin to clear all the glucose produced by high carbohydrate meals from the bloodstream, and their blood sugars will remain at abnormal levels all the time.

If insulin resistance at the muscles and liver is your only problem and you have not inherited abnormal genes that affect your beta cells, over time you may be able to grow new pancreas islets filled with new beta cells. These will secrete and store the huge amounts of extra insulin you need to use for your first- and second-phase insulin releases. This is what happens to a lot of obese people who are often very insulin resistant but never become diabetic.

It is precisely because most people *can* grow new beta cells, even when their blood sugar rises into the prediabetic range, that most people with prediabetes don't deteriorate past the prediabetic stage to full-fledged diabetes.

Unfortunately, when you have impaired glucose tolerance, there is no way of knowing for certain if your rising blood sugars are due solely to insulin resistance and can be handled by growing more beta cells or if they are due to a more worrisome cause: failing beta cells.

Inadequate Beta Cells

Insulin release also fails when beta cells don't secrete insulin normally. This can happen along with insulin resistance or without it. It may be inborn or may develop over the course of your lifetime.

Many gene variants found in people with Type 2 Diabetes cause marginal beta cell function. If your beta cells aren't working properly, they will have to work full-time just to keep up with the need for a basal insulin release. This keeps them from storing any excess insulin in granules for later release. When you are younger you may be able to get along fine with marginal beta cells, but as you get older, anything that makes you need more insulin than usual, like pregnancy, obesity, or normal aging, can lead to secretion failure. Exposure to the many environmental toxins that damage beta cells can also cause or worsen secretion failure, a subject we will discuss further in Chapter Three.

Some people's beta cells may be capable of secreting insulin normally, but fail to do so because something has damaged the their ability to sense that blood sugars are rising after meals and that insulin needs to be secreted. This can be due to defects in any one of several genes within the beta cell that govern this process.

Yet another reason for failing beta cells is autoimmune attack. A subset of people diagnosed with Type 2 diabetes turn out to have a recently discovered slow-developing form of autoimmune diabetes called **LADA** (Latent Autoimmune Diabetes of Adults). In this form of autoimmune diabetes beta cells die off gradually rather than all at once, which is what they do in the more familiar Type 1 form of auto-immune diabetes that is usually diagnosed in children. We will discuss LADA more fully in Chapter Thirteen.

Infections, toxic chemicals, pesticides, and some pharmaceutical drugs can also kill or cripple beta cells even in people who were born with completely normal ones. And though it is a rare cause for diabetic blood sugars, pancreatitis and/or undetected pancreatic tumors will also cause beta cells to stop secreting insulin.

Rising Blood Sugars Further Damage Beta Cells

Whatever the reason for your failing insulin release, there's an ugly feedback mechanism that kicks in as your blood sugar rises after meals. It turns out that high blood sugar itself is toxic to beta cells, a phenomenon called **glucose toxicity**. So as your blood sugar rises, for whatever reason, it causes further damage to your beta cells, which makes your second-phase insulin release even less able to lower your blood sugar.

Rising Blood Sugars Increase Insulin Resistance

When your blood sugar is routinely going over 180 mg/dl, another bad thing happens. Your cells become insulin resistant *even if they weren't insulin resistant before*. So the higher your blood sugar, the more insulin it takes to lower it. The reason for this is that a gene that makes your muscles respond to insulin is shut off by high blood sugar levels. This is a protective mechanism meant to keep high levels of glucose from flooding into your cells and damaging them. Fortunately, this gene will start working again when you lower your blood sugar.

The Fasting Blood Sugar Death Spiral

When the beta cells are no longer able to secrete enough insulin to keep fasting blood sugar normal, it often means you have suffered a critical amount of irreversible beta cell death. When this happens, blood sugar control can deteriorate very swiftly. Remember how we explained earlier that the liver interprets a low insulin level as a sign that blood sugar is low? When the beta cells no longer provide a steady basal insulin release, the liver takes it as a sign that blood sugar is low and then, no matter how high your blood sugar might be, the liver dumps more glucose into your bloodstream.

This effect may explain why fasting blood sugar tends not to deteriorate slowly and steadily but often takes a sudden upward surge of 50 mg/dl or more around the time a person has become diabetic enough for a doctor to notice it and give a diagnosis.

How Many Beta Cells Have to Die to Ruin Blood Sugar Control?

This question was answered by a series of autopsies a team of researchers led by Dr. Peter Butler performed on pancreases taken from Mayo Clinic patients whose medical histories were known. They found that the pancreases of obese patients who had had normal blood sugars had 50% *more* beta cells than those of non-obese normal people. This demonstrated that they had been able to grow new beta cells when they were needed.

Obese patients who had had impaired fasting glucose had lost about 40% of their beta cell mass. Patients diagnosed with fully diabetic fasting blood sugars had 63% less beta cell mass than normal people—which the researchers attributed to beta cell death, not to any shrinking in the size of the beta cells. There was more evidence of recent beta cell death in lean people with diabetes than in obese people with diabetes.

But this is not entirely bad news, as it tells us that even after a diagnosis of prediabetes or diabetes, most people—especially those who are obese—still have a significant number of beta cells remaining. This is the main *functional* difference between Type 2 Diabetes and Type 1 Diabetes. People with Type 1 Diabetes usually have lost nearly *all* their beta cells due to an autoimmune attack.

And the good news is that if you have even a third of your living beta cells left, it is a lot easier to regain control, because there are effective strategies you can use take the strain off those remaining beta cells and help them do their job.

Chapter Three
What Really Causes Diabetes?

Get Rid of the Guilt!

Before we discuss how you can normalize your broken blood sugar metabolism, there's something we need to get straight: You did not cause your diabetes through reckless overeating and criminal laziness.

Despite everything you have read in the media and contrary to what your doctor may have told you, diabetes is *not* caused by obesity. You did not give yourself diabetes thanks to gluttony and sloth.

Because the media have publicized the toxic myth that people with diabetes are responsible for their plight, we're going to take a few moments now to examine what scientists have learned about the real relationship between diabetes and obesity and why *it is much more likely that your diabetes caused your obesity than the other way around.*

A Toxic Myth That Harms People with Diabetes

You have probably already been brutalized by the many statements that appear in the media to the effect that people with diabetes are diabetic because they are lazy gluttons.

These statements might have shamed you into ignoring early warning signs that your blood sugar was not normal. If so, you are not alone. The fear of being labeled a self-destructive glutton frightens many people into avoiding the early diabetes diagnosis that could completely eliminate all diabetic complications.

Once you were diagnosed, these media pronouncements may have filled you with self-hatred that made it all the more difficult to cope with your new diagnosis The belief that faulty behavior caused your diabetes leads to depression, self-loathing, and feelings of helplessness. If you think you are a rotten slob whose moral weakness gave you this crummy disease, you aren't likely to believe you have the ability to prevent further decline.

Even worse, the belief that people with diabetes have brought their disease on themselves inclines doctors to assume that since their diabetic patients did nothing to prevent their disease, they won't make the effort to control it—a belief that leads many to give patients with diabetes substandard care—which is precisely the kind of care most surveys show doctors *do* give to people with diabetes—care that ensures people with diabetes will end up with the tragic complications that shorten their lives and fill their declining years with suffering.

The myth that diabetes is caused by overeating also hurts the one out of five people with Type 2 Diabetes who are *not* overweight. Because doctors only think "Diabetes" when they see a patient who fits the stereotype—the obese, sedentary patient—they often neglect to check people of normal weight for blood sugar disorders, even when they show up with such classic symptoms of high blood sugar as recurrent urinary tract infections, fungal complaints, or neuropathy.

Where Did This Toxic Myth Come From?

Because most people who are obese are insulin resistant—including the two thirds of obese people who do *not* ever develop diabetes—the conclusion was drawn years ago that the insulin resistance seen in people with Type 2 Diabetes was caused by their obesity. It made sense. Something was burning out the beta cells in these people, and it seemed logical that it must be the stress of pumping out huge amounts of insulin, day after day, to meet the needs of the obese, insulin resistant body.

Some studies also showed that substances secreted by fat cells seemed to increase insulin resistance. This reinforced the idea that the insulin resistance seen in people with Type 2 diabetes was caused by their obesity.

This is why it is common for doctors to tell a patient who has just been diagnosed with diabetes that their diabetes was caused by their obesity and that if they could lose as little as ten pounds they would no longer be diabetic—though, as most people with diabetes who have lost ten or even fifty pounds and remained diabetic will tell you, this is almost never true.

But doctors who believe that diabetes could be easily reversed if people would only stop stuffing themselves with food often feel about people with diabetes the way they do about those smokers who refuse to stop smoking even after they develop lung cancer. They consider them a waste of their valuable time, since these patients almost always fail to lose weight and thus, they believe, persist in their self-destructive lifestyles.

With an attitude like this, it's no surprise that many doctors don't keep up on diabetes research. They don't take seminars about the latest ways to treat diabetes. They save their energy to treat patients they think of as more deserving. So because they remain ignorant about what science has learned over the past two decades about the real causes of diabetes, they reinforce the self-hatred of their diabetic patients and don't challenge the media when they repeat misinformation and suggest that diabetes is the punishment fat people bring on themselves for being lazy gluttons.

Even though that belief is completely untrue.

Genes Not Obesity Cause Type 2 Diabetes

While people who have diabetes are often heavy, one out of five people diagnosed with Type 2 Diabetes is thin or of normal weight. And though the CDC reported that slightly more than one out of three Americans was obese in 2010, they also reported that only 20.7 million people out of the entire 311.7 million American population had been diagnosed with diabetes in 2011. That is roughly only 7 out of every hundred. This implies that fewer than one in ten of all those considered overweight actually get diabetes. The others, though they may develop insulin resistance and prediabetes, are very unlikely to develop full-fledged diabetes.

There is a reason for this. Academic research is making it increasingly clear that people who do develop diabetes do so because they have damaged genes. Some are inherited, but others are caused by exposure to a host of chemical toxins that pervade our environment.

Unless you have these damaged genes, you can eat until you drop and though you may get very fat and develop quite a few other health problems, your blood sugar control will stay functional and you will *never* develop full-fledged diabetes.

Twin Studies Back Up a Genetic Cause for Diabetes

Studies of identical twins were the first to suggest that there are genetic causes for diabetes. They found that twins have an 80% concordance for Type 2 Diabetes. In other words, if one twin has Type 2 Diabetes, the chances that the other twin will also get it are four out of five. In contrast, studies of fraternal twins found *no* such concordance. Even when they are raised by the same caregivers and fed the same diets there is a much lower likelihood that two fraternal twins will develop diabetes. Since identical twins have identical genes while fraternal twins do not, this points to a genetic cause, rather than bad habits.

The List of Genes Associated with Diabetes Keeps Growing

Scientists have discovered a long list of genes that interfere with the normal mechanisms the body uses to regulate blood sugar. These are the genes found in people diagnosed with diabetes. Some of the abnormal genes found to be associated with Type 2 Diabetes in people of European extraction include: TCF7L2, HNF4-a, PTPN, SHIP2, ENPP1,

PPARG, FTO, KCNJ11, NOTCh3, WFS1, CDKAL1, IGF2BP2, SLC30A8, JAZF1, and HHEX.

People from non-European ethnic groups have been found to have entirely different diabetic genes, like the UCP2 polymorphism found in Pima Indians and the three Calpain-10 gene polymorphisms found associated with diabetes in Mexicans. There are unique diabetes genes found in people living in Middle East and in the Japanese. Population-specific genes that contribute to diabetes in African Americans have also been identified.

Researchers are also finding that the longer they study a group of subjects over a period of time, the more powerfully the presence of these genes predicts who will get diabetes. They do so far better than the classic risk factors like obesity and a family history of diabetes.

These diabetes genes also become more powerful when found in association with other diabetes genes. One study has found that the more diabetes genes an individual carries, the higher their likelihood is of developing diabetes.

Of great interest, also, is the finding that most of the gene defects researchers have associated with diabetes, including the most common one, TCF7L2, do not cause insulin resistance. What they do is limit the ability to secrete insulin.

Genetic Insulin Resistance May Be Present Before Obesity Arises

Though most diabetes genes appear to cause insulin deficiency, a few powerful and common diabetes genes do cause insulin resistance, and when these genes are active, people are insulin resistant long before they become obese, suggesting that obesity is a result of insulin resistance, rather than the cause.

A revealing study took two groups of *thin* subjects with normal blood sugar who were evenly matched for height and weight. The two groups differed only in that one group had close relatives who had developed Type 2 Diabetes, suggesting they were more likely to have diabetes-related genes. The other group had no relatives with Type 2 Diabetes.

The researchers measured the subjects' insulin resistance and discovered that the thin relatives of the people with Type 2 Diabetes already had much more insulin resistance than did the thin people identical to them in height and weight who had no relatives with diabetes.

Mitochondrial Dysfunction Is Found in Lean Relatives of People with Type 2 Diabetes

The reason for this insulin resistance in people with diabetes genes was made clear by a second, landmark, 2004 study that looked at the cells of "healthy, young, lean" but insulin-resistant relatives of people with Type 2 Diabetes.

The study found that in some thin people who had relatives with Type 2 Diabetes, the mitochondria, which are the parts of the cell that actually burn glucose, appeared to have a defect. While the mitochondria of people who had no relatives with diabetes burned glucose well, the mitochondria of the people with an inherited genetic predisposition to diabetes were not able to burn off glucose as efficiently. Not only that, but this mitochondrial flaw caused the glucose they could not burn to be stored in their cells as fat, which would make it very easy for them to become obese as they grew older.

Some Diabetes Genes Make Exercise Ineffective

Research has also found that a subset of people with diabetes have a specific form of genetic damage that keeps their muscles from being able to burn glucose properly during exercise. This is particularly common in children diagnosed with Type 2 diabetes. Their diabetes turns out not to be the result of "lifestyle choices" or poor parenting, as you might believe if you read media reports, but of having been born with damaged mitochondria.

Insulin Resistance Precedes Weight Gain and May Cause It

Rather than being the result of weight gain, it is starting to look like insulin resistance is a major cause of it. A study that used a new imaging technology compared the energy usage of lean people who were insulin resistant with that of lean people who were insulin sensitive. These researchers found that lean but insulin resistant subjects converted the glucose that came from high carbohydrate meals into triglycerides—i.e. fat. In contrast, lean insulin-sensitive subjects stored that same glucose in the form of glycogen—the storage form of carbohydrate found in muscles and the liver. The researchers concluded that "the insulin resistance, in these young, lean, insulin resistant individuals, was independent of abdominal obesity and circulating plasma adipocytokines, suggesting that these abnormalities develop later in the development of the metabolic syndrome."

Translated into English, what this means is that *people become insulin resistant before they become fat.* More importantly, it says that their insulin resistance was not, as is often claimed, caused by the chemicals given off by fat cells, because they didn't have these fat-related chemicals in their bloodstreams. If they became fat, it was because of the metabolic flaw that led these people to store glucose from high carbohydrate meals as fat rather than in the form of easy-to-burn glycogen, as people not fated to develop diabetes would have done.

The Environmental Factors that Stress Beta Cells and Lead to Diabetes

However, since twin studies show that both identical twins do not always develop diabetes, scientists know that additional factors beyond the presence of an inherited gene may be needed to bring out diabetes in people with susceptible genes. Scientists call these **environmental factors**. Quite a few studies hint at what the environmental factors are that might lead a person who is already carrying the genes that limit the ability to secrete insulin to develop full-fledged diabetes.

A Mother's Diet During Pregnancy May Cause Diabetes

Researchers following the children of mothers who had experienced a Dutch famine during World War II found that children of mothers who had experienced famine were far more likely to develop diabetes in later life than a control group from the same population whose mothers had been adequately fed. The genes of fetuses that are malnourished appear to undergo what are called "epigenetic changes" — permanent non-inherited gene alterations, that make it easier to become diabetic as they age.

This may not seem all that relevant to Americans whose mothers have not lived through famines. But when you consider how many American teens and young women suffer from eating disorders and how prevalent crash dieting is in the group of women most likely to get pregnant this begins to look like it could be a significant factor for some of us.

It is also significant that until the 1980s obstetricians routinely warned pregnant women against gaining what is now understood to be a healthy amount of weight. When pregnant women started to gain weight, doctors often put them on highly restrictive diets that resulted in their giving birth to underweight babies whose low birth weight suggests that they were starved in the womb.

A Mother's Gestational Diabetes May Cause Diabetes

Maternal starvation is not the only pre-birth factor associated with an increased risk of diabetes. Several studies have shown that having a well-fed mother who suffered gestational diabetes also increases a child's risk of developing diabetes.

It is known that a child who inherits a known diabetes gene from their mother is more likely to express that gene more severely than if they inherit the identical gene from their father. This is probably because a mother carrying strong diabetes genes is very likely to have a diabetic pregnancy.

Disruptions of Sleep Patterns and Shift Work Cause Diabetes

It had long been believed that people who work the night shift or who suffer from sleep disturbances develop raised insulin resistance. But in 2012 scientists associated with Harvard University described experiment that challenged this belief.

They exposed normal people to 3 weeks of sleep restriction (5.6 hours of sleep per 24 hours) combined with circadian disruption (recurring 28-hour "days.") They found that this disrupted sleep pattern raised blood sugar significantly both immediately after a meal and in the fasting state.

But the reason for these elevated blood sugars turned out *not* to be rising insulin resistance. Instead it was decreased insulin production. By the end of three weeks, three of the previously normal subjects had developed prediabetic blood sugars.

The weight gain that had been attributed to insulin resistance turned out to be due to the fact that the subjects in the study experienced an average 8% drop in their resting metabolic rates. This, the researchers explained, could lead to a 12.5 lb weight gain over the course of one year.

Toxic Chemicals in Our Environment Also Cause Diabetes

But the above causes only explain a small part of what pushes people with iffy genes into developing full fledged diabetes. A far more important cause is the large number of poorly regulated, dangerous chemicals that pervade our air, water, and food supply.

Pesticides and PCBs in the Bloodstream Correlate with the Incidence of Diabetes Independent of Weight

A study conducted among members of New York State's Mohawk tribe found that the odds of being diagnosed with diabetes in this population were almost four times higher than normal in members who had high concentrations of PCBs in their blood serum. Even worse was the incidence of diabetes in those with high concentrations of pesticides in their blood. This relationship held true regardless of their weight.

This phenomenon isn't limited to people of Native American heritage. A study published in 2009 tracked how much exposure a group of pregnant Belgian woman had had to several common pollutants. It found a correlation between exposure to PCBs and DDE in the womb and a child's developing obesity by age 3. These toddlers' obesity — which may well turn into diabetes — was clearly not due to "lifestyle choices."

Trace Amounts of Arsenic in Urine Correlate with a Dramatic Rise in Diabetes

A study published in 2008 found that, in a group of 788 adults, those who had the most arsenic in their urine were nearly four times more likely to have diabetes than those with the least. High levels of arsenic often result from exposure to industrial coal burning or copper smelting. Exactly how arsenic might contribute to the development of diabetes is unknown, but prior studies have found that an arsenic compound can impair insulin secretion in beta cells. Arsenic is found in almost all rice.

Other Chemicals Cause or Increase Insulin Resistance

The Common Herbicide Atrazine Causes Insulin Resistance

A study published in April of 2009 mentions that "There is an apparent overlap between areas in the USA where the herbicide, atrazine (ATZ), is heavily used and obesity-prevalence maps of people with a BMI over 30."

It found that when rats were given low doses of this pesticide in their water, "Chronic administration of ATZ decreased basal metabolic rate, and increased body weight, intra-abdominal fat and insulin resistance without changing food intake or physical activity level." In short the animals got fat even without changing their food intake. When the animals were fed a high fat, high carbohydrate diet, the weight gain was even greater. It appears that atrazine produces these effects by causing mitochondrial dysfunction, which causes cells to convert glucose to stored fat rather than burn it for fuel.

Another common herbicide, 2,4-D, causes elevated blood sugars through another mechanism. Scientists at New York's Mount Sinai Hospital discovered that the intestine has receptors for sugar identical to those found on the tongue and that these receptors regulate secretion of an important hormone, GLP-1, which we will discuss later in Chapter Nine. In 2009, these scientists reported that the herbicide 2,4-D blocked this taste receptor, effectively turning off its ability to stimulate the production GLP-1. When GLP-1 levels drop, blood sugars rise.

Other chemicals detected in human bloodstreams have been linked to endocrine disruption, obesity, and insulin resistance. Some of these toxins appear to cause permanent genetic damage that can be passed on to children.

Among these are flame retardants and the nonstick compounds that are used both in cooking pans and to make upholstery fabrics stain resistant. A Danish study found that daughters of mothers with the highest concentrations of one of these chemicals, PFOA, in their blood during pregnancy were three times as likely to be overweight at the age of about 20 years as were daughters of mothers with the lowest PFOA blood levels.

Other common chemicals with similar effects are the phthalate plasticizers found in soft plastic goods including food and cosmetic containers. The amount of phthalate allowed in consumer goods is supposed to be federally regulated, but in 2013, when scientists took a selection of common children's toys to the lab, including a Dora the Explorer backpack, they discovered that the actual level present was as high as 69 times the federally permitted limit. Phthalates have been shown to increase insulin resistance in teenagers.

Bisphenol-A (BPA), a plastic previously used in hard plastic goods and dusted on cash register receipts, suppresses a key hormone, adiponectin, which helps regulate insulin sensitivity in the body. This puts people at a substantially higher risk for metabolic syndrome. Though manufacturers have replaced BPA with a different substance, BPS, further research has revealed that this substitute is just as toxic. Like the nonstick compounds discussed above, BPA (and probably BPS) have been shown in animal research to cause damage to offspring exposed to it in the womb, making them more insulin resistant and glucose-intolerant.

Most disturbingly, some evidence has emerged that the damage caused by these toxic substances, including BPA, is passed on to the grandchildren of those exposed, making it clear that these substances permanently alter genes.

Lastly, it's worth noting that no testing has ever been done to see what the effect is on blood sugar and body weight of being exposed to several of these chemicals at one time. All research and resulting regulations consider only the level of a single chemical in isolation.

Prescription Drugs Cause Diabetes

Industrially produced pollutants are only one kind of chemical that can cause diabetes. It turns out that Type 2 Diabetes can also be caused by chemicals we introduce into our bodies on purpose, in the form of pharmaceutical drugs. The highly respected Women's Health Initiative study found that women without diabetes who were taking statins at the start of the 15 year long study had almost twice the risk of developing diabetes as those who were not. Another epidemiological study published in the Journal of the American Medical Association found that people taking high dose statins were 12% more likely to develop diabetes than those taking lower doses. This may occur because statins can limit the ability of the mitochondria to burn glucose.

Other drugs that have been shown to cause diabetes in people who would not otherwise get it include prednisone, beta blockers, and atypical antipsychotic drugs including Zyprexa and Abilify.

It is also likely that the SSRI antidepressants, which are known to cause obesity, promote diabetes. For years, the companies that make these drugs explained the higher rates of diabetes seen in the population taking these drugs by claiming that people with diabetes are more depressed than the population at large. But a study published in 2008 tested this hypothesis against the huge population studied in the Diabetes Prevention Program (DPP) trial. It found that "a strong and statistically significant association between antidepressant use and diabetes risk in the PLB and ILS arms was not accounted for by measured confounders or mediators."

In English, this means that having depression previous to taking the drug did not correlate to a heightened risk of getting diabetes, only taking an antidepressant did.

Treatment for Cancer, Especially Radiation, Greatly Increases Diabetes Risk Independent of Obesity or Exercise Level

A study published in August 2009 analyzed data for 8,599 survivors in the Childhood Cancer Survivor Study. It found that after adjusting for body mass and exercise levels, survivors of childhood cancer were 1.8 times more likely than their siblings to report that they had diabetes. Even more significantly, those who had had full body radiation were 7.2 times more likely to have diabetes.

How Diabetes Really Develops

Now that we have a better understanding of the underlying physiological causes of diabetes, let's look more closely at the physiological processes that take place as people become diabetic and learn the real relationship between obesity and diabetes.

As we've seen, people destined to develop diabetes are often born with genes that limit their ability to secrete insulin. Often these genes occur along with others that increase insulin resistance. Toxic exposures then further increase their insulin resistance and damage their beta cells. Some toxins even create new, heritable diabetes genes.

Rising Blood Sugars Increase Insulin Resistance

Over time, people who have only a marginal ability to secrete insulin combined with insulin resistance, whether inborn or caused by toxic exposures, begin to experience a slow rise in their post-meal blood sugars. Then one of the nastiest features associated with rising blood sugar occurs. As these post-meal sugars rise, they make it easier for blood sugar levels to rise even higher.

This is because when blood sugars cross a threshold in the upper part of the range most doctors consider to still be normal—a level somewhere between 160 and 180 mg/dl—they cause **secondary insulin resistance** to develop. This is a new kind of insulin resistance that is distinct from the inborn insulin resistance we discussed earlier. This new secondary insulin resistance worsens any previously existing insulin resistance.

Researchers have discovered why this happens. It turns out that normal people have a "fat-burning" gene that secretes an enzyme which is needed to maintain the cell's insulin sensitivity. But the expression of this gene is reduced in the muscle tissue of people who are experiencing high blood sugars. So lacking the enzyme that is made by this gene, muscles develop reduced insulin sensitivity and impaired fat burning ability.

Then, at a certain point, these rising post-meal blood sugars reach a level that is high enough to kill beta cells. In a normal person, who has the ability to grow new beta cells, any damaged beta cells will be replaced by new ones that will secrete enough insulin to keep their blood sugar low enough to avoid further damage. But as we explained at the end of the previous chapter, the beta cells of a person with the kinds of damage we're discussing seem to be unable to reproduce. Perhaps the rate at which beta cells are being killed is too high for new beta cells to replace those that died, or perhaps when blood sugars reach a certain threshold, glucose toxicity keeps the cells from reproducing normally. Whatever the explanation, these people's blood sugars spend hours every day at the elevated levels that kill off their already compromised beta cells.

Rollercoaster Blood Sugars Cause Overeating

Many readers may still be thinking, "Don't tell me about genes. I got fat because I overate." And no one is saying you didn't. But what you may not realize is that the reason you overate was almost certainly because as your blood sugars rose to abnormal levels after meals, due to the processes we just described, you developed the so-called "roller coaster blood sugars" that are known to cause relentless hunger.

This happens long before a person is diagnosed with diabetes or even with prediabetes, at the time when first-phase insulin secretion has started to fail. For people with weak first-phase insulin secretion, eating a meal rich in carbohydrates will send blood sugars soaring high above normal for at least an hour after eating. But because at this early stage of blood sugar deterioration you still have a very strong second-phase insulin release, these levels plummet back to normal quite swiftly over the next hour. When your blood sugar drops this way it causes a relentless, nagging hunger, which can make you obsessed with food.

The reason for this has to do with the fact that your brain requires a certain amount of glucose to stay alive. Just a few minutes of very low blood sugars can put you into a coma. So as soon as your blood sugar starts plunging down, your brain sends out messages that cause hormones to rise in a way that floods you with the feeling that if you don't eat some carbohydrates — right now — you're going to die. It's meant to keep you safe. Unfortunately, it makes you fat!

It's important to note that your blood sugars don't have to drop into the range doctors consider hypoglycemic to cause this kind of relentless hunger. Any steep, fast drop in blood sugar, even one that ends in the normal range, will do it.

But since doctors consider you "normal" if your two hour glucose tolerance test result is under 140 mg/dl, a doctor will see nothing unusual about a blood sugar that rises to 199 mg/dl one hour after eating and plummets to 99 mg/dl half an hour later, even though that 100 mg/dl steep drop is enough to convince your brain you're heading for a dangerous low blood sugar, which will cause it to go into high alert and send out "Eat more carbs, now!" messages that leave you ravenous.

This explains why, as your blood sugar control deteriorated, two hours after you ate a high carbohydrate meal you may have ended up hungrier than you were before you began eating. If you responded by eating more carbs, you provoked another blood sugar spike that led to another steep drop that made you even hungrier. Over time, this kind of blood sugar rollercoaster may have pushed your eating completely out of control.

But your problem wasn't a moral failure, it was physiological. Blood sugar swings are a known problem with a known cure. But most doctors don't attribute obesity to this kind of hunger because they are taught that intense hunger only occurs when blood sugars drop into the official hypoglycemic range — below 70 mg/dl. When you show up in their offices with a weight problem and blood sugar that, if it tests abnormally at all, is likely to test slightly high, your doctor does not connect your overeating to those rollercoaster blood sugars.

Instead, if you tell your doctor you are experiencing overwhelming hunger, they may suggest that you have an emotional problem and give you an antidepressant — which will worsen your insulin resistance. Or, if you're a middle aged female, you may be told that your sudden and terrifying weight gain is a common menopausal symptom, which will abate in time.

But here's the good news. Once you know that you have a blood sugar abnormality, be it prediabetes or full-blown diabetes, your days of misery, hunger, and out of control eating are over. Not because you are going to turn into a better person and rediscover some hidden source of will power, but because there are well-understood ways of dealing with a broken blood sugar metabolism that can flatten out your blood sugar, eliminate that hunger, and free you from the domination of blood sugar swings.

And you don't have to lose a single pound make it happen!

Chapter Four
Blood Sugar Level and Organ Damage

Before we can teach you how to restore your blood sugars to normal levels we need to settle the question of what levels truly *are* normal. The obvious answer is that normal blood sugar levels are those that don't cause the terrible organ damage doctors describe with the euphemism "diabetic complications."

Surprisingly, there is very little medical research directed at answering the question of what those levels might be. Almost all the diabetes-related research you see reported in the medical news is research about the benefits of this or that new drug. Since none of the diabetes drugs lower blood sugar very much, these studies are careful to avoid connecting the blood sugar levels these drugs produce with the incidence of complications.

The studies that do connect blood sugar levels to organ damage rarely make their way into the medical press. To find them, you must comb through obscure journals published for academic researchers. But the information is there, buried in studies performed by scientists from different disciplines using many different research techniques. Surprisingly, all these studies point to a narrow range of blood sugars as being where the various diabetic complications begin.

In this chapter, we'll summarize what these studies tell us about what blood sugar levels cause organ damage. If you want to read the actual research papers, you'll find the citations in the Reference section at the end of this book. You can also find links to many of these studies online at **Bloodsugar101.com,** along with relevant new studies published since this book was published.

Blood Sugar Level and Nerve Damage

Neuropathy is a word that means "sick nerves," and nerve damage is one of the earliest and most devastating diabetic complications. Neuropathy appears to strike when blood sugars remain over 140 mg/dl for two hours or more.

Because nerves start to become damaged at the "mildly" elevated blood sugar level most doctors ignore, almost one half of people with Type 2 Diabetes already have detectable neuropathy by the time they are diagnosed with diabetes. Many other people who are *never* officially diagnosed with diabetes but who have higher than normal blood sugars also get "diabetic" neuropathy.

The pain of neuropathy usually starts in your feet. It can feel like tingling or burning, though some people describe it as feeling like there is something stuck between their toes when there really isn't anything there.

Diabetic neuropathy differs from the nerve pain that can be caused by disc problems in the back in that it usually is symmetrical—i.e. it occurs in both feet. Less commonly, diabetic neuropathy can cause problems in the hands and arms.

Nerves affected by neuropathy eventually become numb. When you are examined after your diabetes diagnosis, your doctor should test your feet with a tuning fork or a thin filament that looks like fishing line to see if you have dead nerves in your feet that you may not have noticed. Many people with diabetes do. It is an important finding that tells the doctor you have a high risk for developing serious infections.

Neuropathy Affects More than Just Your Feet

While the nerves of your feet are the ones you are most likely to notice, the presence of neuropathy in your feet suggests that other nerves in your body are also under attack, including the nerves of the autonomic nervous system, which control functions like blood pressure, heartbeat, sexual response, and the movement of food through your digestive system.

Research has found that the more years you spend with high blood sugars, the more likely you are to develop sexual dysfunction. Nerve damage often explains the presence of erectile dysfunction that can't be corrected with Viagra and similar drugs. Neuropathy also leads to gastroparesis, the condition where food stays in your stomach for many hours because the nerves controlling the stomach valves don't work properly.

Another nerve that gets damaged by high blood sugars is the vagus nerve, a vital nerve that connects your brain to the rest of your body. The vagus nerve has been found to play a major role in the regulation of the immune system. Neuropathic changes in the vagus nerve may have something to do with why people with diabetes have trouble fighting infections, since a weakened vagus nerve may not signal the immune system that your body is under attack.

The vagus nerve also regulates heartbeat. It is possible that damaged vagus nerves may have something to do with the high incidence of fatal heart attacks in people with diabetes. Abnormal heartbeats may also contribute to sudden cardiac death.

Neuropathy is painful, which is bad enough, but if it is allowed to progress, eventually it can lead to amputations. This happens partially because the death of nerves keeps the immune system from sensing and responding to infections and partially because what kills your nerves is the failure of the tiny blood vessels that supply them with nutrients. When your blood sugar is high for a long time, glucose clogs these tiny vessels and compromises blood flow. Nerves die from lack of nutrients and oxygen, and germ fighting cells can't reach the infected tissue. If the blood vessels in your limbs get clogged badly enough, a simple infection may lead to your developing gangrene.

Doctors don't have any effective treatment that reverses neuropathy. Instead, they offer psychoactive drugs that limit your ability to feel the pain. This relief, while welcome, doesn't prevent the nerve damage from continuing.

Neuropathy Correlates Closely to Post-Meal Blood Sugar Levels

So what has science found about the blood sugar level at which neuropathy starts to develop?

A lot. Several studies run by neurologists at different clinics discovered that the incidence of neuropathy starts to rise significantly in people whose blood sugar two hours after an oral glucose tolerance test is 140 mg/dl or over—i.e. people with prediabetes.

Neurologists at The University of Utah found that patients who were not known to be diabetic, but who registered readings of 140 mg/dl or higher on a two hour glucose tolerance test, were much more likely to have the diabetic form of neuropathy than were those who had lower blood sugars. Even more telling, the researchers found that *the length of time* a patient had experienced this nerve pain correlated with how high their blood sugar rose over 140 mg/dl on the glucose tolerance test.

What was also interesting about this study was that it found *no* correlation between the incidence of neuropathy and the two blood sugar tests most doctors who treat diabetes rely on to evaluate patient health. *Neuropathy did not correlate to any particular fasting blood sugar level, nor did it correlate to any particular A1c value.* But in people whose blood sugars were higher than 140 mg/dl two hours after they drank 75 grams of glucose there was a sudden significant increase in the incidence of diabetic neuropathy.

A second study performed by neurologists at Johns Hopkins confirmed these findings. Fifty-six percent of their patients who had neuropathy of unknown origin were found to have abnormal results on their oral glucose tolerance tests. The neurologists investigated the nerve damage further and learned that patients whose OGTT results fell in the prediabetic range had suffered damage to their *small* nerve fibers. The fully diabetic subjects whose OGTT results were over 200 mg/dl had more damage to their *large* nerve fibers. Yet another study, conducted at the Mayo Clinic in Scottsdale, AZ and published in August 2006 confirmed these results.

Anecdotally, many people who post about their experiences with diabetes on the web have reported that they can make the pain in their feet go away by keeping their blood sugars under 140 mg/dl at all times, though if they let their blood sugar rise, the pain will come back. Typically it takes three to six months for these lower blood sugars to produce results. Some of those who control their blood sugar tightly also find Alpha Lipoic Acid and Benfotiamine helpful for healing their nerves. We will discuss both in Chapter Eleven.

Blood Sugar Level and Serious Illness

High blood sugars make you more prone to infection. So it is worth noting that a study found that when doctors kept the blood sugars of seriously ill hospitalized patients below 140 mg/dl at all times they improved their survival. A doctor working in an acute care setting was able to decrease the death rate of a group of critically ill patients by 29.3% simply by using insulin to keep their blood sugars below 140 mg/dl at all times.

This intervention also cut down the incidence of kidney failure and shortened the patients' stay in the ICU. This means that 45 people out of a group of 800 left the hospital alive who would have died had their doctors adhered to the ADA's recommended target of 180 mg/dl, which is how they define "tight control."

Blood Sugar Level and Beta Cell Dysfunction

Beta cells turn out to be very sensitive to slight rises in blood sugar. In fact, there's some evidence that beta cell dysfunction may begin when blood sugar spends more than a few hours at levels over 100 mg/dl.

A team of Italian researchers studying how the beta cells of normal people responded to rising glucose discovered that a small amount of beta cell dysfunction began to be detectable in people whose blood sugar remained only slightly over 100 mg/dl at two hours after the start of a glucose tolerance test. The higher a person's blood sugar remained the more beta cells were failing.

Another study found that beta cells start to die off in people whose *fasting* blood sugar is over 110 mg/dl. But this finding may be misleading. Remember how in Chapter Two we learned that fasting blood sugar doesn't rise to 110 mg/dl until post-meal blood sugars have been high for several years? That makes it likely that it is not their mildly elevated fasting blood sugars that are killing these people's beta cells, but the much higher post-meal blood sugars that are occurring when their fasting blood sugar has reached that level. These studies did not test their research subjects' post-meal blood sugars.

Which brings us back to the question of how high does blood sugar have to rise to kill a beta cell?

In mice, the answer seems to be over 150 mg/dl. Normal and diabetic blood sugar levels in rodents are the same as they are in people, though there are important differences in how rodents metabolize glucose, which explain why scientists have cured mice of diabetes hundreds of times without coming up with anything that works in humans.

In mice, exposure to blood sugar concentrations over 150 mg/dl killed transplanted beta cells that were previously healthy. Researchers working with mice receiving beta cell transplants showed that beta cell death was much lower in groups of mice receiving beta cell transplants whose blood sugar was kept under 150 mg/dl than it was in those who were allowed prolonged exposure to blood sugars higher than 150 mg/dl.

But you're a man, not a mouse! Even so, it doesn't matter. A series of experiments done with cultured human cells found that prolonged exposure to high blood sugars kills human beta cells too, and the higher the glucose level the beta cells were exposed to, the more dysfunctional they became.

They also discovered that there was a *time threshold* beyond which the damage to beta cells caused by exposure to elevated blood sugars became irreversible. The researchers took cells that had been damaged by exposure to high blood sugars and moved them to media that had a lower concentration of glucose. They found the cells could survive and recover after being moved to a growth medium containing a much lower concentration of glucose, but *only if the switch was made before a certain amount of time had passed*. Once the cells had been exposed to glucose for that fatal time period, they could no longer be revived.

Though the study did not cite the specific blood sugar level at which damage occurred, I emailed the author of this study who wrote back, "I think the glucose toxic effects begin when blood glucose gets above 140 and probably earlier."

Blood Sugar Level and Retinopathy

Retinopathy means "sick retina" and it is among the most terrifying of diabetic complications. The retina is the part of the eye that contains the nerves that transmit light images to the brain. What happens in retinopathy is that after extended exposure to high blood sugars the tiny blood vessels that feed the nerves of the retina become clogged. In response, a great number of fragile new blood vessels start to grow throughout the retina in a disordered manner.

These disordered diabetic blood vessels have weak walls, unlike healthy vessels, and eventually they burst, releasing blood into the eye. Fluid may leak into the macula, the part of the retina that produces sharp, central vision. This causes a dangerous condition called macular edema. Left untreated, these overgrown vessels may eventually destroy the optic nerve's ability to transmit images to the brain, resulting in permanent blindness.

It's important to note that retinopathy has no symptoms. The blurry vision some people experience when their sugars rise is not from retinopathy but from sugar entering the fluid in the eyeball and changing its optical properties.

Doctors currently treat retinopathy by using lasers to zap shut bleeding or swollen blood vessels in the eye. This helps retain vision, though it cannot restore nerves that have been destroyed by the blood vessel overgrowth. Expensive new drugs, monoclonal Anti-VEGF antibodies, can also be helpful in treating macular edema.

"Diabetic" Retinopathy is a Prediabetic Complication

It was long believed that diabetic retinopathy did not develop until blood sugar levels on the OGTT were well over 200 mg/dl. It was because they held this belief that the American Diabetes Association's experts chose 200 mg/dl as the blood sugar level to be used to diagnose diabetes. Unfortunately, as is the case with so many of the theories the ADA's experts relied on to determine what blood sugar levels were safe, this turned out to be wrong.

One major study of a large population of people with prediabetes discovered retinopathic changes in the eyes of one out of every 12 people diagnosed with *prediabetes*. Even more significantly, these people developed "diabetic" retinopathy even when they did *not* go on to develop blood sugars high enough to be diagnosed as diabetic.

Another study, the French DESIR study of people diagnosed with prediabetes, found that subjects who developed retinopathy over a nine year period had an average fasting blood sugar of 130 mg/dl and an average A1c of 6.4%. Those who did *not* develop retinopathy over this period had an average fasting blood sugar of 108 mg/dl and an average A1c of 5.7%. They did not measure post-meal values.

A meta-study, published in late 2010, based on the records of "44,623 participants aged 20 to 79 years with gradable retinal photographs" found that the incidence of diabetic retinopathy rose significantly as soon as one of the following happened: fasting blood sugars rose to the 115-122 mg/dl range, glucose tolerance test 2-hour results reached the 176 – 191 mg/dl range, or the A1c rose into the 6.3-6.7% range. These are all levels that most doctors would currently label "prediabetic."

The good news, if you have been diagnosed with early retinopathy, is that, just as was the case with neuropathy, lowering your blood sugar can improve your retinal health. Some people who lower their blood sugars will experience a temporary worsening in their retinas when they first begin lowering their blood sugar. Even so, follow-up of one major study, the Diabetes Control and Complications Trial (DCCT), found that, ten years after they had begun to lower their blood sugar, patients who developed early worsening had similar or more favorable outcomes than those who did not lower their blood sugars, even though those who did not lower their blood sugars did not experience this early worsening.

Blood Sugar Level and Cancer

Cancer cells have to eat, and glucose is their favorite food. Therefore it should come as no surprise that cancer rates rise significantly in people with "mildly" impaired blood sugars.

A Swedish study that followed 64,597 people for 10 years discovered that there was a large increase in the risk of cancer for those participants, no matter what their weight might be, who had fasting blood sugars over 110 mg/dl or who scored over 160 mg/dl two hours after a glucose tolerance test.

The risk continued to grow as participants moved into the diabetic category, but it did not increase by the same increment as it did when they moved from normal to what most doctors consider only "mildly" impaired.

The cancers that responded the most strongly to exposure to higher blood sugars appear to be those of the pancreas, endometrium, urinary tract, and malignant melanoma.

Blood Sugar Levels and Heart Attack

It has long been known that people with diabetes have a higher risk of having a heart attack than does the rest of the population. But, as was true with other "diabetic" complications, it turns out that the actual risk of having a heart attack begins to rise when blood sugars are near the top of the normal range and doubles at blood sugar levels considered to be *prediabetic*.

Not only that, but if you are wondering about your own risk of heart attack, it turns out that your post-meal blood sugar levels predict the possibility of heart attack much more reliably than do your cholesterol test results.

Most people believe that high cholesterol predicts heart attack risk because this idea was promoted very heavily to market the expensive statin drugs that lower cholesterol. But it turns out that fully one half of all people who have heart attacks have normal cholesterol. Among those who have heart attacks who do have high cholesterol, analysis of the Framingham Heart Study data shows clearly that it isn't their LDL or total cholesterol levels that predict heart attack. It is their triglyceride levels and their ratio of total cholesterol to HDL.

A recent study found that triglycerides are stored in abnormal amounts in heart muscle very early in the progress of diabetes, when blood sugar levels have risen only slightly over normal. What raises triglycerides? Dietary carbohydrates. What improves the ratio of total cholesterol to HDL? Lowering carbohydrates. The oral diabetes medication metformin also significantly lowers triglycerides. Statins don't.

Post-Meal Blood Sugars Predict Carotid Artery Wall Thickening

Insight into why blood sugar might be so closely related to heart attack incidence was given by a study published by an Italian team in 2008. They reported that in a group of people with diabetes who were measuring their blood sugar at home the increase in the thickness of the carotid artery wall over five years correlated directly with how high their blood sugars rose after meals.

One Hour OGTT Result over 155 mg/dl Correlates with Markers for Cardiovascular Disease

A second study published in 2009 gave glucose tolerance tests to people whose blood were sugars considered normal (under 140 mg/dl at two hours after the start of the test) or prediabetic (under 200 mg/dl at two hours). It linked blood sugar readings one hour after ingesting glucose with two more markers that are associated with subclinical inflammation: high fibrinogen and a high white blood cell count. Those readings were also associated with abnormal lipid ratios and insulin sensitivity. It concluded that a one hour GTT blood sugar over 155 mg/dl could be considered a new marker for cardiovascular risk.

A1c Accurately Predicts Heart Attack Risk

As we've mentioned, few doctors pay any attention to post-meal blood sugars. But it also turns out that the A1c is a far better predictor of heart attack risk than are cholesterol levels. This astonishing finding was discovered during a large-scale study called EPIC-Norfolk. What's particularly valuable about this study is that the researchers conducting it weren't looking for the causes of heart disease. They were studying cancer. Their finding that A1c predicted heart disease in people with supposedly normal blood sugar was a shocker.

Here's the summary from their published conclusions:

> In men and women, the relationship between hemoglobin A1c and cardiovascular disease (806 events) and between hemoglobin A1c and all-cause mortality (521 deaths) was continuous and significant throughout the whole distribution. The relationship was apparent in persons without known diabetes. Persons with hemoglobin A1c concentrations less than 5% had the lowest rates of cardiovascular disease and mortality.

In addition, the researchers concluded, "These relative risks were independent of age, body mass index, waist-to-hip ratio, systolic blood pressure, serum cholesterol concentration, cigarette smoking, and history of cardiovascular disease." In short, it wasn't weight or cholesterol that mattered. Blood sugar and blood sugar alone predicted whether or not a person was likely to have a heart attack.

Another study, which drew similar conclusions, discovered an even tighter correlation between A1c and heart disease risk that began as A1c rose above 4.6%, a level that is thought to correspond to an average blood sugar level near 86 mg/dl. This study found that the risk of heart attack doubled for every 1% rise in A1c. So a person with a 5.6% A1c had double the risk of someone with a 4.6% A1c.

However, before you interpret this to mean that you are doomed, it is important to realize that "risk" is a statistical concept that exaggerates small differences. It is illuminating to ignore "risk" and look at the actual incidence of the heart attacks reported in the EPIC-Norfolk study. As Table 3 shows, for every 100 men, there were 5 more cardiac "events," i.e. heart attacks, when the A1c of the group rose from 5% to 6%, but for women there was only an additional one and a half cardiac events per hundred when the average A1c of the group rose by that amount. The published study notes that only slightly more than 20% of these cardiac events were fatal. This suggests to me that the 5% A1c range, which most people with diabetes can attain without undue struggle, greatly improves our chances of avoiding a fatal heart attack.

Why A1c Correlates to Heart Disease Risk

An intriguing study published in 2011 may explain both why measuring cholesterol gives such confusing correlations with heart disease and why the A1c does a better job of predicting it. It found that LDL becomes dangerous when it becomes glycated—i.e. when sugar molecules become bonded to it—because when that happens LDL is more likely to stick to the artery walls.

Since the A1c actually measures the glycation of red blood cells, it may well be a good index to how much glucose has become bonded to other proteins in the blood, including LDL.

Sexual dysfunction has long been known to correlate with the same kinds of vascular changes that cause heart disease. Though there is surprisingly little research into the relationship between blood sugar level and sexual dysfunction, several studies have found a link between rising A1c levels and an increase in erectile dysfunction that echoes the connection between A1c and heart disease.

A1c	<5.0%	5-5.4%	5.5-5.9%	6.0-6.4%	6.5-7.0%	>7.0%	Known Diabetes
Number of Men	1204	1606	1153	374	84	81	160
Coronary Events per 100 men	3.8	6.4	8.7	10.2	16.7	28.4	21.9
Number of Men's' Events	46	102	100	38	14	23	35
Number of Women	1562	1967	1378	439	73	68	83
Coronary Events/100 women	1.7	2.1	3.0	7.3	9.6	16.2	15.7
Number of Women's Events	26	41	41	32	7	11	13

Table 3. Actual Heart Attack Data from the EPIC-Norfolk Study

Does Normalizing A1c Reduce Cardiac Risk or Raise It?

Two large studies published within weeks of each other in early 2008 came to dramatically different results on this question. Sadly, because most doctors have time only to read the headlines and don't look into the details of these studies, many patients are being given the toxic — and inaccurate — advice to keep their A1cs high to protect their hearts.

The first published study, called ACCORD, found that a population of people with diabetes and heart disease who had followed an aggressive program of lowering blood sugar had slightly *more* heart attack deaths than a control group who strove for higher targets, even though the group who followed the aggressive program attained an average A1c of 6.4%.

However, the second study, ADVANCE, which had enrolled twice as many subjects as ACCORD and lasted longer, found *no* increase in deaths in the group of participants this study treated more aggressively. They too attained an average A1c of 6.4%.

Subsequent analyses of the ACCORD data revealed what it was that was to blame for the very slight increase in mortality in the group shooting for lowered A1cs: high blood sugars. Though people in the ACCORD "tight control" group were shooting for lower A1cs, many in that group did not achieve them, and it was the people with *high* A1cs in that group who appear to have had a higher risk of death.

As one analysis concluded, *"Higher average A1C was associated with greater risk of death."* [emphasis mine] A principle investigator for one site involved in the ACCORD study is also quoted as saying,

> An A1c below 7% alone does not appear to explain the excess deaths in the ACCORD trial and is not necessarily a predictor of mortality risk. ... Further, the rate of one-year change in A1c showed that **a greater decline in A1c was associated with a *lower* risk of death.**

The Heart-Toxic Drugs Avandia and Actos Were Also to Blame

There are many different ways to lower A1c—but in both these studies patients eating high carbohydrate/low fat diets controlled their blood sugars entirely through the use of antidiabetic drugs. Which drugs were used varied from study to study. Supplementary material published with the ADVANCE study, the one which found no increase in deaths in the group that lowered A1c, shows that ADVANCE relied mostly on the sulfonylurea drug, Gliclazide, which as we will see later, in Chapter Eight, is a safe drug that doesn't harm the heart. Unfortunately, it is not sold in the United States.

Patients in ADVANCE who did not get to goal with Gliclazide were put on metformin and several other drugs including basal and fast-acting insulin. But only 32 (.6%) of the 5,571 people in the intensive control arm of ADVANCE were taking Avandia or Actos.

The case was very different in ACCORD. 4,702 of the 5,128 people in the intensive treatment arm of ACCORD were taking either Avandia or Actos—and 91.7% of those were taking Avandia. As you'll read in Chapter Eight, it is now known that that both Avandia and the similar drug, Actos, cause heart failure.

Another bit of information that got lost in the reporting about ACCORD is that the full text of the research paper makes it clear that the increased risk of excess death in the tight control group was largely found in people who had *already* experienced heart attacks before the study started—those who would have been most prone to the heart failure Actos and Avandia promote. Among those who had not had heart attacks before the study, the risk of heart disease *dropped* with tight control.

If your doctor warns you that lowering your A1c below 6.5% raises the risk of heart attack, share these findings with him—the citations can be found in the Reference section of this book. And remind your doctor, too, that both ADVANCE and ACCORD found that lowering A1c lowered the incidence of the classic diabetic complications—neuropathy, retinopathy, and kidney disease.

Blood Sugar Levels and Stroke

The risk of stroke also rises as blood sugars rise. The Whitehall prospective cohort study that tracked 19,019 men for 38 years found that their risk of death from stroke increased 27% with a 18 mg/dl rise in their glucose tolerance test two hour result.

The researchers found that as the subjects' two hour glucose tolerance test result rose above 83 mg/dl, their risk of stroke rose in a linear fashion, meaning that the higher their blood sugar at two hours, the more risk of stroke. Though again it's important to remember that the calculations used to estimate "risk" inflates the resulting percentage. The actual prevalence of fatal stroke in this total population over the 38 year period was only 6.5%.

Blood Sugar Levels and Kidney Disease

Kidney failure is a common and devastating diabetic complication that condemns the sufferer to dialysis unless they are fortunate enough to get a kidney transplant. A study published in 2004 that followed 1,871 adults with diabetes for 11 years as part of the Atherosclerosis Risk in Communities Study found that the risk of developing serious kidney disease rose significantly as soon as the A1c rose over 6.0% and increased in a straight line manner as the A1c climbed higher.

So once again, it looks like "diabetic" kidney disease begins to occur at prediabetic blood sugar levels.

But there is more to the story than just how high blood sugars rise. It turns out that blood sugar *fluctuations* cause more damage to kidney cells than do steady state high blood sugars.

A study done on kidney tissue found that exposing kidney cells to blood sugar levels that fluctuated between 135 mg/dl and 270 mg/dl did more damage to those cells—in terms of causing the growth of fibrous tissue—than did constant exposure to high blood sugars. The researchers who published this study explain that it is not glycation (the attachment of glucose molecules to proteins) that destroys the kidney tissue so much as the effect of the fluctuations of blood sugar on the expression of various genes.

The authors of this study concluded, "These results ... imply that important differences in end organ damage could occur in individuals with similar HbA1c but different postprandial glucose levels." They urge that more attention be paid to eliminating large blood sugar spikes.

Blood Sugar Levels and Tendon Problems

Though many doctors are not aware of this, tendon problems appear to be yet another diabetic complication. Carpal tunnel syndrome and frozen shoulder (adhesive capsulitis) are two common tendon problems that are found at much higher rates in people with diabetes than they are in the general population. Dr. Richard K. Bernstein, the noted diabetes expert, has written that he also considers iliotibial band syndrome (closely related to piriformis syndrome) to be a little known diabetic complication. Piriformis syndrome is an entrapment syndrome where a nerve that passes down the hip into the leg gets compressed and causes sciatic pain. As you will no longer be surprised to hear, these conditions too, appear to occur more frequently in people whose blood sugars are in the prediabetic range. For example, one study that analyzed a patient database found that 71.5% of those diagnosed with frozen shoulder had been diagnosed with either diabetes or prediabetes. The percentage of those with the condition who had a prediabetes diagnosis was 33%, not much lower than the 39% who had been diagnosed with diabetes.

Another study found that among people diagnosed of prediabetes, a diagnosis of carpel tunnel syndrome was a good predictor of a diabetes diagnosis ten years later. This is particularly significant as we have seen that most people with prediabetes do not go on to develop full-fledged diabetes. Though carpal tunnel syndrome was attributed by the researchers in this study to the nerve damage caused by high blood sugar, it is just as likely that its real cause is the thickening of tendons that other research has found to be common among people with diabetes. This thickening was seen to grow worse with increasing age in people with diabetes, though not in the general population.

The underlying reason for this thickening may be that tendons have a sparse blood supply and so may be among the very first tissues to experience early vascular damage in the presence of even slightly higher than normal blood sugars. Dr. Bernstein suggests that glycosylation of tendon or muscle tissue may also be at fault.

There is also some interesting academic research connecting degenerative disc disease to elevated blood sugars. The vertebral discs of people with degenerative disc disease rupture, resulting in damage to the nerves that exit the spine. This can cause chronic pain and, in some cases, paralysis. Research into the connection between blood sugar and degenerative disc disease has identified several important structural changes in the disc material of rodents and/or people with diabetes that weaken the tissue, making it prone to rupture. In a slightly different kind of study, researchers conducted glucose tolerance tests in men whose necks had been x-rayed and found that ossification [hardening into bone] of two major ligaments in the neck was more frequently found in those with both "diabetes or impaired glucose tolerance."

Unfortunately, the most common treatment for both tendon conditions and disc-related pain is cortisone, administered via a shot or a course of prednisone pills. These treatments may actually hasten the progression from pre- to full-fledged diabetes, because cortisone therapy not only worsens blood sugar during the week after the therapy—something doctors are aware of—but can also leave some people with blood sugars that remain permanently higher than they were before the cortisone treatment. Doctors are not aware of this, but many of us who are active online have experienced this permanent worsening after taking prednisone, including myself.

This is not only tragic, but unnecessary, as studies have found that cortisone treatments do not improve the healing of tendon problems. In fact, some research has documented that, in patients with frozen shoulders, cortisone treatment may actually produce a *worse* long-term outcome. But even so, most doctors still prescribe cortisone shots or pills as a placebo, perhaps so that their patients will feel that they got something in return for their expensive visit beyond the advice to be patient and let time do its work.

The Safest Blood Sugar Levels Are . . .

The data we've reviewed so far seems to point to A1cs in the lower 5% range and post-meal blood sugars between 140 and 150 mg/dl as being the highest safe levels. Above those levels heart disease and neuropathy begin to become more common, as do tendon problems. Kidney damage appears to begin when A1cs approach the 6% range and blood sugars are spiking very high after meals. Retinopathy becomes more frequent when A1cs reach the low 6% range,

This is probably why the American Association of Clinical Endocrinologists (AACE) currently recommends that people with diabetes try to keep their blood sugars under 140 mg/dl as much as possible. Sadly, the American Diabetes Association still tells people with diabetes that a blood sugar level of 180 mg/dl two hours after eating is "tight control" and suggests that this level is all people with diabetes need ever strive for.

Clearly, the lower you can get your blood sugar, the better, but A1cs in the 5% range and post-meal blood sugars that stay under 140 mg/dl as much as possible appear to be good enough. These are levels that many people with Type 2 Diabetes are able to attain. Many in the online diabetes community who have maintained at those levels for years have not developed the classic complications, and if they had complications at diagnosis, they have not progressed and may even have reversed.

If you have been running very high blood sugars for a while, lowering your blood sugar to a safe level may seem like a daunting task. But don't worry! All people with diabetes can do far more than most doctors realize to lower their blood sugars, and most can bring their blood sugars down into the safe range using the techniques we'll be discussing in Chapters Six through Ten.

Frequently Asked Questions about Blood Sugar Levels

When people decide to lower their blood sugars, they often have questions about how exactly they should be measuring them. Those questions generate much of the mail that I get from visitors to my web site. Here are the answers to the most common questions people ask me.

What If A1c Results Conflict with Meter Readings?

People who measure their blood sugar at home frequently ask why their A1cs are higher than would be expected based on meter testing. They worry that even though they are keeping their post-meal readings in the normal range their risk of complications is still high.

It isn't. It turns out that the A1c test, though useful when applied to large populations, can fail when estimating an individual's blood sugar. The formula used to estimate average blood sugars from A1c readings were derived from a population whose average A1c was well above 7.0%. These formulas sometimes fail when applied to people whose blood sugars are near normal. The A1c test assumes that red blood cells live only three months. But some research suggests that red blood cells live longer when blood sugars are normal, and, of course, the longer a red blood cell lives, the more glucose it will accumulate, which raises the A1c—even in the presence of normal blood sugars. At the other extreme, as we have mentioned, if you are anemic or have certain inherited blood conditions that affect red blood cells, your A1c may be *low* when your blood sugar has been spiking high after meals.

Other, unknown genetic factors may also be involved. Studies have shown that some people's A1cs are consistently higher than their blood testing would suggest while others' are always lower—and that these differences persist from test to test. So if your A1c predicts an average blood sugar that does not correlate to your blood sugars as measured after many meals, trust the post-meal measurements. It is most likely that they, not your A1c, predict complications.

Are Isolated High Fasting Blood Sugars Dangerous?

People also often wonder how dangerous their high fasting blood sugars might be if they are keeping their post-meal readings normal. Many people report that no matter what they do or how normal their blood sugars are after eating, their fasting blood sugars are their highest of the day.

This is not unusual and is due to something called "dawn phenomenon." What happens is this: your body prepares for waking up by secreting several different hormones. First, between 4:00 and 6:30 a.m. it secretes cortisol, epinephrine, and norepinephrine. You may recognize these as the hormones involved in the "fight or flight response." In this case, their job is more benign, to give you the energy to get up and moving.

To give you this burst of energy, these hormones raise your blood sugar. Around 5:30 a. m., after these stress hormones have raised the blood sugar, a normal person's insulin starts to rise. But people with diabetes don't have a normal relationship with insulin, so instead of getting a small shot of morning energy that is quickly metabolized they get an abnormally high fasting blood sugar.

If you are injecting insulin or taking a drug that stimulates insulin secretion, another reason you may be seeing surprisingly high fasting blood sugars may be that your blood sugar is dropping abnormally low while you sleep. When this happens your body will secrete stress hormone to push your blood sugar up to a safe level. If increasing your insulin dose or oral medication makes your blood sugar go up rather than down, this may be the explanation.

Yet another reason for higher than expected fasting blood sugars is taking too much blood pressure medication. Abnormally low blood pressures will also provoke a release of stress hormones that not only raise blood pressure but also blood sugar.

If this is your problem, changing the time of day when you take your medications can sometimes help. If you inject long-acting insulin, ask your doctor if you can split your dose into a larger morning and smaller evening dose to avoid late night hypos. You also can try using Levemir or the new basal insulin, Tresiba, rather than Lantus.

The good news is that many studies have found that elevated fasting blood sugars that aren't accompanied by high blood sugars after meals don't correlate strongly with the likelihood of developing complications. So if you find that your fasting blood sugar is the highest of the day, though you control your blood sugar very well during the rest of the day, there is no reason to stress about it.

When Exactly Should You Test After Eating?

When the topic of testing blood sugar one or two hours after a meal comes up, people often asks when they should start measuring those hours. Should it be the beginning of the meal or when they have finished eating? The question is particularly worrisome for those who take their time eating their meals.

There is no one-size-fits-all answer here. When we test after a meal, what we are really interested in seeing is how high the highest reading is that resulted from meal. For many people this will occur about an hour after the start of the meal. But other factors besides leisurely dining can affect when that spike occurs. Individuals can digest foods at slightly different speeds, especially those who have had diabetes long enough that it has affected the nerves that control digestion. In addition, meals high in fat may cause the carbohydrates they contain to digest more slowly.

There is no need to obsess about this. If you are unsure when your own blood sugar peaks after eating, test a couple meals at fifteen minute intervals starting at one hour after your first bite. You will soon see when your actual peak occurs and can then test those meals only at the time you would expect to experience that peak.

Why Don't We Test Before One Hour?

If you test your blood sugar half an hour after the beginning of a meal, you will often see a higher reading than the one you find when you test at any other time. This raises the question of why research seems to ignore those peaks.

The answer is that blood sugar spikes that resolve before an hour has passed after eating don't appear to harm to our organs or even raise our A1cs. It takes a period of time for blood glucose to permanently attach to and damage the proteins that make up our organs. A brief fifteen minute blood sugar spike doesn't appear to last long enough to let this happen.

Chapter Five
Must You Deteriorate?

The Toxic Myth Your Doctor Believes

When you start to use the strategies you'll read about in the next couple chapters, wonderful things happen to your blood sugar. You stop experiencing the blood sugar swings that were making you hungry or crazy, you lose a couple pounds without trying, and you start to feel good. A month later, you realize that your blood sugar is finally low enough that, if the research cited here is right, maybe you won't have to lose your feet like Grandma did or go blind like Uncle Willy. Then, just when everything is going so well, you make the terrible mistake of confiding your enthusiasm to your doctor—who tells you not to get your hopes up, because no matter what they do, everyone with diabetes always deteriorates.

Congratulations. You've just run into the second toxic myth that kills and maims people with diabetes.

This toxic myth is the single most dangerous idea that you are likely to encounter as you begin your struggle to live a healthy life with diabetes. It is the belief that science has proven, beyond a doubt, that no matter what you do, your Type 2 Diabetes will get worse.

Your doctor almost certainly believes this. Though he may give lip service to the idea that you can control your disease through diet, exercise, and drugs, what he really believes is that nothing you can do will make much difference in your long-term outcome. This is why your doctor doesn't urge you to lower your blood sugar to normal levels, but merely writes you prescriptions for drugs that, at best, do a mediocre job of controlling your blood sugar. After all, why should he urge you to struggle and deprive yourself of treats when the truth is that no matter what you do, you're doomed?

There are several reasons why doctors believe this. Some will tell you that they've seen it in their practices. They'll tell you that they've treated lots of patients with Type 2 Diabetes and that few, if any, of their patients can achieve anything near normal blood sugars with diet or, for that matter, with all but the most dangerous drugs. They'll add that though they have counseled their patients to lose weight, their patients don't, and even those who have good control end up with complications.

If you challenge the doctor further, he's likely to tell you that it isn't just his patients, the research shows *everyone* with diabetes deteriorates regardless of how good their control might be and to back this up he will cite the one big study that doctors always cite when the topic of good control for people with Type 2 Diabetes comes up, the UKPDS.

Did the UKPDS Prove People with Good Control Still Deteriorate?

The **UKPDS** (United Kingdom Prospective Diabetes Study) was the largest, most exhaustive research study ever run to investigate what happens when people with Type 2 Diabetes improve their blood sugar control. It was an attempt to duplicate another landmark study, the **DCCT** (Diabetes Control and Complications Trial), which was a study of people with autoimmune *Type 1 Diabetes*, which found that people with Type 1 Diabetes who maintained tight blood sugar control got far fewer diabetic complications than those with higher A1cs. Unfortunately, when it was complete, the UKPDS appeared to prove that tight control had far fewer benefits for people with *Type 2 Diabetes*.

Doctors will tell you that the UKPDS proved that the A1c test results of even the patients with good control gradually worsened every year. Not only that, but the UKPDS found that good control only made a small difference in the rate of complications, and that over the course of the study even the people with good control got lots of complications.

This was best exemplified in a Continuing Medical Education (CME) presentation by a distinguished English diabetes expert, Dr. Roy Taylor, a professor of medicine and metabolism at the University of Newcastle upon Tyne. It is no longer available online, but when it was, viewers could see this well-known diabetes expert point to a chart taken from UKPDS data titled "Newly Diagnosed Type 2 Diabetic Subjects Showing Progression of Retinopathy" and explaining,

> These data are usually presented as showing a wonderful difference between the groups, [those controlling their blood sugar and those not] a 37% relative risk reduction. But take another look. This slope is unfortunate. This slope is almost equally unfortunate for the individuals concerned. Although intensive therapy in Type 2 Diabetes over 15 years makes a difference, it's not a staggering difference.

Later when he discusses the UKPDS findings about the progression of nerve damage he says "the abnormal nerve function continues to progress inexorably." When discussing early signs of kidney damage, he delivers the same message. "Intensive therapy [i.e. blood sugar control] does not seem to be able to stop this."

So it is no surprise that Doctor Taylor concluded that controlling blood sugar in Type 2 Diabetes may make a small difference,

> ... but not such a huge difference that you would want to go out of your way as a patient to achieve it, perhaps, if you were shown this graph and told that over 15 years of intensive therapy you would be not much different compared with a "laissez faire" approach.

In short, this doctor is saying you might as well eat that donut, because no matter what you do, you're going to go blind.

Abandon Hope All Ye Who Enter Here?

If Dr. Taylor was right, logic suggests that you might as well enjoy that slice of cake while you can still see well enough to find your fork. If there is nothing you can do, it is rational behavior to shift your energy elsewhere and enjoy life—including the foods you love—while you can.

But in fact, this is *not* true. Doctor Taylor and his peers missed one extremely important point in considering the UKPDS data.

Based on the findings of the research we reviewed in the previous chapters, *"Good Control" as defined in the UKPDS study was really mediocre control.*

Why? Because the definition of "good control" that was used in this study and, indeed, almost every study ever published, defined "good control" to mean that patients achieved A1cs of 7.0%.

When we apply the formula used at the time of the UKPDS study to determine what average blood sugar corresponds to the 7.0% A1c the UKPDS defined as "good control," we quickly see why the UKPDS "good control" group is getting all those complications.

That 7.0% A1c mapped down to an average blood sugar of 172 mg/dl.

But because the A1c reflects only the *average* blood sugar and gives us no idea of the blood sugar *range*, the average blood sugar value any formula comes up with is deceptive. It can't distinguish between the person whose average blood sugar level of 172 mg/dl was achieved by maintaining their blood sugar at a steady 172 mg/dl throughout the day and the person who achieved that average with a blood sugar that surged up to 300 mg/dl, stayed there for two hours, and then plummeted to 70 mg/dl. Since the people in UKPDS were urged to eat a high carbohydrate/low fat diet and given large doses or insulin or drugs that stimulate the production of insulin, it is almost certain most of them were experiencing a pattern of very high blood sugar peaks followed by valleys.

So rather than proving that "good control" doesn't prevent complications, the UKPDS only proved that an average blood sugar of 172 mg/dl, achieved by getting daily post-meal readings that may be going well over 200 mg/dl, is toxic. Which you knew already.

Think of it this way: How would you feel if your doctor said that most patients who quit smoking develop lung cancer—after defining "quit smoking" as "smoked only seven cigarettes a day?"

A Lesser-known Study Got Better Results than UKPDS

As we mentioned earlier, the A1c an indirect measurement that is used to estimate an average blood sugar. It ignores the very important question of how high blood sugars are spiking after meals. So what happens if instead of measuring only the A1c, you measure post-meal blood sugars and attempt to control how high they go?

A ground-breaking Japanese study of people with Type 2 Diabetes who were using insulin answered this question definitively. The researchers in this study, which was conducted in Kumamoto Japan, found that by lowering post-meal blood sugar targets they were able to keep the A1cs of participants stable over the study's entire six year course. Instead of the "inevitable decline" in A1c and blood sugar control that was seen in the UKPDS, the people with Type 2 Diabetes in the Kumamoto study saw *no deterioration at all*.

Not only that, but over the course of the study, the incidence of retinopathy, kidney damage, and nerve damage was dramatically lower in the group that maintained tight control. That group as a whole also saw slight improvements in their neuropathy by the end of the study rather than the deterioration seen in all other studies.

What makes this study so interesting is that the average A1c of the people in the Kumamoto "intensive intervention group" was *identical* to the average A1c of the people in the UKPDS study. What was different was that the blood sugar control strategy the Kumamoto study used focused *on keeping post-meal blood sugars lower*. So the Kumamoto study showed that *preventing high post-meal blood sugar spikes resulted in a much better health outcome, no matter what the resulting A1c.*

This is extremely good news for people who do not wish to succumb to inevitable decline. Especially since the patients in the Kumamoto study were aiming for a relatively high peak of 180 mg/dl after meals.

That is low enough to decrease secondary insulin resistance, but it is still much higher than the blood sugar level that should eliminate most diabetic complications.

A 2006 Study Proved Not All Type 2s Deteriorate and Some Even Improve

A long-term study of people with Type 2 Diabetes run at the Mayo Clinic measured the C-peptide levels of people with Type 2 Diabetes every two years over a period of twelve years. C-peptide is a substance found in the blood that can be used to estimate how much insulin a person is still making. Here's what they found:

> Insulin secretion ... declined with increasing duration of diabetes in approximately half of the patients *but either increased or remained essentially constant over time in the other half* ... These data indicate that although a decrease in insulin secretion over time is characteristic of Type 2 Diabetes mellitus, it is not inevitable.

It is a shame they didn't tell us more about those people whose insulin production didn't decline or improved. Were they shooting for lower post-meal blood sugar targets? Eating a certain diet? Hitting the gym? Bowling? And did their insulin production increase because their insulin resistance was decreasing or because there was less stress on their beta cells? Without this information the study is not as informative as it might be. But like the Kumamoto study, it certainly answers the question, "Do I have to deteriorate?" with a resounding, "No!"

All those Studies that Claim People with Diabetes Get . . .

Along the same lines, once you are diagnosed with diabetes, you will notice a steady stream of depressing stories in the media that report on studies that supposedly prove that people with diabetes are more likely to get everything from cancer to corns.

When you read these articles, remind yourself that almost every participant with diabetes in these studies had an A1c above 7.0% — it is usually *because* they have A1cs over 7.0% that they were considered diabetic by the scientists conducting the study — and that the conditions they came down with were not due to a specific disease, diabetes, but to their years of exposure to dangerously high blood sugars.

What Have Studies Learned About People Who Keep Post-Meal Blood Sugars Under 140 mg/dl?

So far, very little, because no such studies have been conducted. When presented with the erroneously reported results of the ACCORD study, which as we explained appeared to suggest that lowering A1c raised the risk of heart attack, many influential doctors concluded that lowering A1c was dangerous. I have even heard from patients whose prescriptions were taken away when their blood sugar began to approach normal levels by doctors who warned them that they must raise their A1c above 6.5%, not lower it. Some have even been told that, because they are over the age of 50, they should keep their A1cs as high as 7.5%. The follow-up studies that debunked the original ACCORD conclusions received little press and few doctors ever heard about them.

As a result, further research into the benefits of lowering blood sugar came to a complete halt. The only evidence we have now comes from members of the online diabetes community who have maintained their health for almost 20 years now. Many of us are now in our 60s and 70s and continue living active lives free of diabetic complications thanks to having joined the 5% Club.

The Choice Is Up to You

Since we can't point to rock solid research that proves that keeping your blood sugar under 140 mg/dl will completely eliminate complications, you might think you are taking a gamble by committing to that approach. But you are also taking a gamble if you don't. So the question you have to ask yourself is, "Which gamble has the highest cost if I'm wrong?"

If you pursue the regimen we recommend in the next chapters and achieve the blood sugar targets that we have suggested to you, and a decade hence some definitive study shows that even with excellent control and normal blood sugar levels patients still deteriorate, all that you'll have lost is a lot of carbohydrate-laden meals—and possibly some weight.

But if you settle for that 7.0% A1c your doctor recommends with its post-meal spikes over 200 mg/dl, and in ten years the studies show that keeping blood sugar under 140 mg/dl at all times *does* prevent most diabetic complications, you will have paid for your choice with bleeding retinas, failing kidneys, and gangrenous toes.

In addition, if following the dietary approach we describe in the next chapter lets you lower your blood sugars to safe levels with few or no drugs, you are less likely to suffer from as the as-yet undiscovered, dangerous, long-term side effects of new diabetic drugs that won't be known for at least a decade.

So before you let your doctor give you a license to slack off, remember what is at stake: *it's not your doctor's retinas, kidneys, and toes that fail if your doctor is wrong.*

Chapter Six
How to Lower Blood Sugar

Now it's finally time to take the steps that will bring your diabetic blood sugars down to the healthy levels that can restore you to normal health.

To do this is a multi-step process. The first step is to **change your diet** by cutting down the amount of carbohydrate you eat. This is the single most powerful tool you have with which to bring your blood sugar down to levels that are low enough to avoid any further damage to your body.

For many people, even those who were found to have extremely high blood sugars at diagnosis, cutting carbohydrates out of their diet is all they need to do to regain their health. In the rest of this chapter we'll explain how you can do this without making yourself crazy, because most of us have found that none of the other steps you can take to achieve normal blood sugars will work if you don't cut back to some extent on your carbohydrate intake.

If you can't attain healthy blood sugars after you've eliminated the high carbohydrate meals that are so toxic to your beta cells, the next step is to work with your doctor to **see if any of the safer diabetes drugs might work for you.** In Chapter Eight and Nine we will explain to you everything you need to know to select such a drug from the list of those available.

If after adding one or two safe diabetes drugs to a diet that keeps carbohydrates under control you still can't get normal blood sugars, the final step, which *always* works, is to ask your doctor to help you craft **a modern insulin regimen.** This is an insulin regimen that restores your basal insulin, as well as, if you need it, your second-phase insulin. Don't shudder when you hear the word, "insulin." In Chapter Ten, we'll calm your fears about insulin and show you why going on insulin early rather than late may be the smartest thing you will ever do for your health.

Harness the Power of an Effective Diabetes Diet

Diet is the most powerful tool you have for restoring your body to normal health. But don't let the dreaded "D-word" fill you with foreboding or feelings of hopelessness. The diabetes diet we are about to describe here has little in common with the restrictive ordeals you may have suffered through in the past in vain attempts to lose weight.

This diabetes diet is not about calories. You are not going to have to starve yourself. You still get to eat dessert. The diabetes diet is not a low fat diet. Nor is it—despite what you may have heard—a high protein diet.

When you get your own personal diabetes diet working, it will do two wonderful things for you: It will lower your blood sugar to a safe level and it will keep you from feeling hungry between meals.

The key words here are "your own personal diet." The diabetes diet that works for you is not necessarily the one that works for me. As we've stressed before, different things are broken in each of our metabolisms. So the goal of this chapter is not to tell you what to eat. Instead, what we are going to do is give you the tools and techniques you can use to design your own personal diabetes diet.

To do this, you're going to rely on three simple tools, your blood sugar meter, the log you will keep of your blood sugar test results, and a good reference that gives you nutritional information for the foods you eat. With these tools you'll be able to determine the exact diet that will make the best use of whatever beta cell function you have left. With these tools, you'll also be able to determine if diet is enough to restore your health or if you should investigate diabetes drugs. If you are taking a diabetes drug, you'll see how well it is controlling your blood sugar. If you exercise, you'll learn how that exercise affects your blood sugar, too.

Using these tools will make you far less dependent on your doctor because you will know exactly how well your blood sugar is doing every day. When you visit your doctor you'll have clear blood sugar goals you want to attain and a good idea of how close you are to attaining them. You'll also be able to determine if your current doctor is willing and able to help you attain those goals or if it is time to look for a new doctor who will give you the support you need.

Your Power Tool: The Blood Sugar Meter

Your blood sugar meter is the single most powerful tool available to undo the damage caused by diabetes. In Chapter Four we reviewed the medical research that suggests that it is high post-meal blood sugars that damage your organs and, over time, lead to nerve death, amputation, blindness, and kidney failure. Your blood sugar meter can help you lower those post-meal blood sugars to the level where they stop damaging your body.

The way your blood sugar meter will do this is by showing you exactly what each meal you eat is doing to your blood sugar. It will help you see which foods are raising your blood sugar to dangerous heights, so you can eliminate them and replace them with other foods you enjoy that don't have that effect.

How to Choose The Right Blood Sugar Meter and Test Strips

Since your blood sugar meter is so important, it is essential to choose one that is both reliable and affordable. You may find very cheap or even free meters at the pharmacy or online. But it is not the cost of the meter that dictates how affordable your testing will be, it's the cost of the **test strips** you must use each time you test your blood sugar. These strips are not reusable and they are extremely expensive.

Over the decade I've been using a meter, I've seen the cost of every other technology plummet to the point where I can buy a brand new computer that has a hundred times the power of my 1998 computer for one fifth of what I paid for that 1998 computer. But the price of test strips just keeps going up. Strips that were $.60 apiece in 1998 are now $1.34, (and up $.29 just since 2008). Worse, they aren't any more accurate now than they were back then. Since you will be doing a lot of blood sugar testing as you learn to lower your blood sugar, it's important to find a meter whose strips are affordable.

In the United States you can buy a blood sugar meter and test strips without a prescription at any drug store. However, if the cost of your meter and strips are going to be covered by health insurance or Medicare, you will need a prescription from your doctor that specifies the exact brand. People covered by Medicare can get one meter of their choice for free. Many private insurers offer selected brands of meters and strips at an affordable co-pay. Often they are one of the name brand meters: LifeScan One Touch, FreeStyle, or Accu-Chek. These are decent meters, and if your insurer will help pay for the strips, take them up on it. But the strips used with these brand name meters are exorbitantly expensive if you have to pay for them yourself. So if you need more strips each month than your insurer will pay for, you might want to buy a second, cheaper meter that uses cheaper strips.

There are some tradeoffs involved in using the cheaper meters. The Relion meters sold by Walmart costs about $9 and the strips it uses cost less than half of what the name brand strips cost. But their quality can vary because the specific meters sold under the Relion brand change from year to year and appear to be made by a variety of manufacturers. I have found that some Relion models are quite good, while others consistently read very high.

Another meter with cheap strips is the TRUEtest meter, which can be bought at many online stores. However, online reviews for this meter often report that they give inaccurate results, though other people find them useful. Drug stores also sell cheaper generic brand meters.

But despite the drawbacks of these cheaper meters, if your insurer limits your access to inexpensive test strips, a cheap meter with cheap test strips will still be of great help in lowering your blood sugar as long as its readings are consistent with each other, even if those readings are consistently higher or lower than lab test results.

The quality of the no-name meters marketed aggressively to people on Medicare by mail order companies is more questionable. Be aware that Medicare will pay for name brand meters and strips if your doctor prescribes them. Medicare Advantage plans may also offer much better coverage for meters and strips than traditional Medicare.

Some people report having good experiences buying name brand strips from sellers on eBay or Amazon. I have done this myself. Just be sure that the expiration date on the strips hasn't passed. And don't order strips online when it is either very cold or very hot, as they may be damaged by exposure to temperature extremes during shipping.

Several companies sell cheap, generic test strips online, which are advertised as being compatible with any older One Touch Ultra meter that allows you to change the meter's code. However, the accuracy of these strips is questionable, with many people reporting that they are inconsistent and that they deliver readings far different from actual One Touch Ultra strips. The FDA issued safety alerts and recalls for both GenStrip and UniStrip generic test strips in 2014, though both can still be purchased online. As attractive as the price might be for these, their questionable accuracy makes them a poor choice for the way you will be using your meter here.

Meters usually come with a lancet device, which is a spring-loaded object that looks like a pen. Its job is to shoot a little needle tip into your finger, just deep enough to draw blood. Some meters also come with a starter set of disposable lancets that fit into the device.

Painless Blood Sugar Testing

If someone who doesn't themselves have diabetes taught you how to test your blood sugar, for example a nurse at a hospital or your doctor's office, they may have taught you the wrong testing technique, one that makes testing unnecessary painful. Here are some tips about how to test painlessly that have been shared by people who have posted on the web over the past decades.

Where to Test

The least painful spot to do a blood sugar test is on the side of your finger. Do not test on the pad of the finger. That hurts!

Many of us find that our pinkies have the best blood flow, but the sides of any but your pointer finger are also good choices.

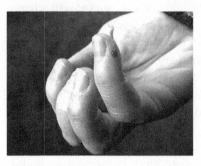

Figure 2. The least painful place to test

Dr. Bernstein, the distinguished diabetes doctor and author who has had diabetes himself since 1946, recommends using the back of the finger, below the base of the nail. For me, that location hurts, so I don't use it. I have also seen the fatty pad at the base of the thumb recommended, but that doesn't work for me, either. The lesson from this is that you will have to try all these different suggestions and choose the one that works for you.

Be sure to adjust the depth of your lancet to the shallowest depth before you test. That is usually "1" on most lancets. If that is too shallow to draw blood, adjust it up one notch and try again. As you get calluses on your fingers from testing, you may need to adjust the depth again. However, once you develop calluses you can keep using the same lancet depth as long as your continue to get enough blood. Once calluses develop, your tests should also become more painless.

What About Testing on Your Arm?

Though many meters now offer the option of testing on your arm and promote this as if it were a benefit, many of us find that testing on our arms is more painful than using the sides of the fingers. And there is another more important problem: When you test your arm rather than your finger tip, the reading you get will lag about 15 minutes behind the reading you would have gotten using your finger tip. This is because the skin in your arm contains more interstitial fluid than your finger tips. It also means arm testing is worthless for detecting the dangerous hypoglycemic low blood sugars often referred to as **hypos**.

Alcohol Toughens Skin

There is no need to dab your skin with alcohol before testing. Dr. Bernstein reports that neither he nor any of his patients has ever developed an infection after testing without alcohol. I have never used alcohol in over 18 years and have never developed an infection from a lancet blood test either.

The use of alcohol over time will dry out and toughen your skin, making it harder to draw blood. If your hand is dirty, wash it. If you see an unexpectedly high reading, you should also wash your hand

and try again. A tiny bit of glucose or sugary food on your finger can cause dramatically high readings.

You Can Reuse Your Lancets

If you are the only person using your lancet device there is no need to use a fresh lancet for each test. I change mine once every few months. Some people report changing theirs even less frequently. Many of us find used lancets are more comfortable to use than new ones.

Less Painful Lancet Devices

Several brands of lancets are marketed as being less painful or even pain-free. I have tested several and found that the Accu-Chek cartridge device is by far the least painful, probably because it has the slimmest needle. These come free with Accu-Chek meters, but you can also purchase them separately at the drug store. Because I change lancets infrequently, one box of cartridges for the Accu-Chek device has lasted me more than 7 years, and I test a lot.

Never Share a Lancet!

If someone else is going to share your lancing device — for example a relative interested in knowing whether their blood sugar is high after a meal — you *must* give them a fresh lancet and dispose of it immediately after they use it to avoid transmitting any blood borne diseases — including those neither of you might know that you have. Never violate this policy!

Disposal of Test Strips

Blood products are considered medical waste. If you don't have access to a red bio-waste container, make one out of an old detergent bottle. When it is filled, tape the top closed and mark the container "Caution: Medical Waste." Then dispose of it according to your local trash ordinances. You can also buy inexpensive medical waste disposal units at most local pharmacies.

Meter Accuracy

There is a lot of misinformation floating around the web about meter accuracy. You will often hear that meters may be off by as much as 20%. This is not true. While the standards that meter companies are required to meet *do* allow them to be off by 20%, in practice the meters sold now by reputable companies are usually much more accurate. Most of the time, when your blood sugar is near 100 mg/dl two meters of the same brand testing a drop of blood from the same puncture should give you a reading that is no more than 5 mg/dl different. At much higher blood sugar levels, the gap may be bigger.

Meters from different companies may give readings that differ from each other by more than that. Anecdotally, people report that Accu-Cheks may give readings a bit higher than do One Touch Ultras.

Two readings taken on the same meter from two different punctures made as little as five minutes apart may also vary by a larger amount because the concentration of glucose in your blood can vary over that interval. To test how consistent your meter is, test the same drop of blood with two different strips using the same meter. If the readings are within 10 mg/dl, your meter is consistent enough to be helpful.

To determine how accurate your meter is, when your doctor schedules you for a fasting blood test, bring your meter along and test right before the blood draw. That way you can compare your meter reading with the lab result. Don't be concerned unless the difference between your meter and the lab is larger than 10%. At readings near 100 that would represent a difference of 10 mg/dl.

Though any hint of inaccuracy is annoying in a device that uses such expensive test strips, for now you'll have to live with it. For the way we will be using our meters, a meter's consistency with itself is the most important thing. If I know that my Ultra always reads 10 mg/dl lower than the lab result when my blood sugar is near 100 mg/dl, I can live with it because what I'm most interested in knowing is how *high* my blood sugar rises after eating or how low it drops after taking insulin or another medication. A consistent meter should portray the size of the rise or fall accurately.

There is no need to waste strips running the control solution test that is recommended by the makers of blood sugar meters. Defective meters often deliver "in range" results with control solution tests. As far as I can tell, the only reason manufacturers include control solution is so that the meter company can claim that almost any meter they sell is accurate. I have gotten "in range" control solution test results even when a comparison with a lab draw showed my meter to be giving readings that were off by 25%.

If you wonder what the best brand might be at any given time, check with people who frequent web diabetes discussion forums. Over time models change, so today's best meter may not be the one most recommended next year.

Meters have moved away from needing you to set a code on the meter to match the code on each new batch of strips. But if you use an older meter that still needs coding, make sure that you have set the meter code to match the strip code before you test. This can make a big difference in accuracy.

Avoid leaving your test strips in a very hot or cold place, like your car, as exposure to temperature extremes may damage them and render previously accurate strips inaccurate.

Once you have obtained a blood sugar meter and practiced using it a few times, you will be ready to start lowering your blood sugar.

Step 1: Set a Healthy Blood Sugar Goal

In Chapter Four you read the scientific evidence that hints at what blood sugar levels damage your organs. Now it's time to commit to lowering your blood sugar below the level where that damage is likely to occur. Table 4 below presents four different sets of blood sugar targets. Each set includes a post-meal blood sugar target, an A1c target, and a fasting blood sugar target. These targets range from the most rigorous to the most lax. Your first step is to choose which blood sugar targets you will be aiming for.

Note that although the chart gives targets for fasting blood sugar and A1c, we will be concentrating almost entirely on lowering our post-meal blood sugars. This is because most of us find that when we lower our post-meal blood sugars enough to attain our post-meal targets we see our fasting blood sugars and A1cs drop into the recommended range.

	CGMS Normal	5% Club	AACE	ADA
1 Hr after meal	120 mg/dl	Under 140 mg/dl	Not Given	Not Given
2 Hrs after Meal	85 mg/dl	Under 120 mg/dl	Under 140 mg/dl	Under 180 mg/dl
A1c Result	4.3% - 5.4%	5.0 - 5.9%	6.5%	7.0%
Fasting Blood Sugar	85 mg/dl	Under 110 mg/dl	Under 110 mg/dl	Under 130 mg/dl

Table 4. A Selection of Post-Meal Blood Sugar Targets

The most rigorous blood sugar targets are the True Normal targets derived from Dr. Christiansen's study, described in Chapter One, which used a continuous glucose monitor to examine the blood sugars of truly normal people. That target matches pretty closely the targets suggested by Dr. Richard K. Bernstein, who was the first to insist that people with diabetes could and should achieve truly normal blood sugars. These are the most rigorous blood sugar targets, and achieving them should eliminate any health problems caused by elevated blood sugars. Their drawback is that they can be extremely hard for people with diabetes to attain unless they adopt very limited, stringent diets.

The next most rigorous set of blood sugar targets are those used by the people in the online diabetes community who call themselves "The 5% Club" because they strive to keep their A1cs in the 5% range. These are the blood sugar targets I shoot for myself. These targets are well below the levels associated with most diabetic complications.

While they may be less than perfect, they are more easily attainable and often won't require that you live a life of stringent self-denial. If you shoot for The 5% Club blood sugar targets you are very likely to end up with an A1c in the 5% range.

The next set of targets, which are even laxer, includes those suggested by the American Association of Clinical Endocrinologists (AACE). If you use the AACE targets you should end up with an A1c near that organization's recommended A1c of 6.5%. These targets come in barely under the levels that research suggests damage organs.

The last blood sugar targets listed are the ones recommended the American Diabetes Association. Using them may result in your achieving an A1c in the 7% range that the ADA considers good enough for people with diabetes. But people with A1cs of 7% still develop a lot of neuropathy, retinopathy, and other diabetic complications.

People often ask me what post-meal blood sugar goal they should shoot for. But I won't tell them. Your blood sugar goals are *your* blood sugar goals, not mine. So you have to decide what blood sugar levels are acceptable. You're the person who has to do the work to reach those goals. You're the person who is going to suffer if they are wrong or who may blow off the whole program if they are too stringent.

If you currently have very high blood sugars, there is nothing wrong with setting a modest goal and celebrating when you achieve it. But after you achieve that triumph, I urge you to review the data in Chapter Four very carefully to see if you would benefit from choosing a more rigorous target going forward.

Step Two: Find Out How Your Current Diet Affects Your Blood Sugar

Now it's time to use your blood sugar meter to determine how high your blood sugar rises after meals when you eat your usual diet. For now, you won't be making any changes to what you eat. All you will be doing is testing your blood sugar after eating several of your usual meals and observing how the foods you are currently eating affect your blood sugar. Here's what to do:

❖ **Measure your blood sugar before your meal**. Note your pre-meal blood sugar reading on a blood sugar log of some type. You can use a smartphone app or the little book that comes with your blood sugar meter. There's no need to be fancy, though. You can also just track your meals using a pad of lined paper. Just note the date and time along with your blood sugar reading. If you use an app, make sure it is flexible enough to let you note which foods you ate at meals and that it lets you track readings taken at times other than before a meal.

❖ **Eat a meal made up of foods you routinely eat**. Note what time it is when you finish eating your meal. Summarize what you ate at this meal. If there isn't enough room to describe your food in your log, write it down somewhere else, or send yourself an email to remind yourself of the menu. It is very important to be able to link the blood sugar reading you obtain after eating a meal with information about what food was in that meal.

❖ **Test your blood sugar one hour after you finished your meal.** Write your blood sugar test result in your blood sugar log along with what time it was when you tested.

❖ **Test your blood sugar two hours after you finish your meal.** Again, write down the results in your log along with the time.

Test a typical lunch and a typical dinner. Then test a breakfast. Do this until you have accumulated test results for six or seven meals you frequently eat.

After you test a few meals, you should start to notice when it is that you experience the highest blood sugar after a meal. For many of us, it's about an hour after eating. But those of us who have slow digestions may see a later peak. And as you will discover, some foods or combinations of foods always digest more slowly than others.

If your access to strips is limited, once you determine when your highest blood sugar tends to occur, you may decide only to test at that time. Or you may alternate between testing at one and two hours.

Learn More About the Foods that Raised Your Blood Sugar

Gather your test results and pick out all the meals that raised your blood sugar over your chosen blood sugar targets. If that's all of them, don't worry. Most people with diabetes will see blood sugar values that are going well over 200 mg/dl after just about every meal. That's why they have been diagnosed with diabetes!

Now take another look at the foods that raised your blood sugars, keeping this important fact in mind: **It is the carbohydrates you eat that raise your blood sugar after meals.** Sugars and starches. Nothing else.

If you have Type 2 diabetes, the fats you eat won't raise your blood sugar at all. Nor will the protein. It is true that protein *can* raise your blood sugar, very slowly, because your liver will sometimes convert about 58% of the protein you eat into glucose, but since it takes up to seven hours for dietary protein to turn into glucose, the only people who experience a slow rise in their blood sugar after eating protein are those whose diabetes is so severe that they have no beta cell function left at all. Most people with Type 2 Diabetes don't see their blood sugar rise after eating protein.

But every gram of carbohydrate you eat, whether it comes from sugar, bread, potato, pasta, fruit, "low glycemic foods," or what the food industry likes to call "healthy whole grains," *does* turn into glucose once it is digested. And as soon as that glucose enters your bloodstream it will raise your blood sugar and cause what we call a **blood sugar spike**. In order to lower those damaging spikes you will need to lower the amount of carbohydrate you eat at each meal.

To be able to do this effectively, you will need to figure out how much carbohydrate there was in the meals that raised your blood sugar to unacceptable heights. Then you will want to learn how much carbohydrate there is in other foods you enjoy eating, looking for those that contain fewer carbohydrates per serving, since these foods would be better choices for your meals going forward.

Even if your testing shows that your blood sugars are completely normal after eating high carbohydrate meals and that you are only diabetic in the fasting state, it's still worth trying out the techniques described below to see if they will lower your fasting blood sugar. This is because it is possible your body is unable to secrete insulin to cover the fasting state because it has to use all the insulin it can make to cover the carbohydrates in those high carb meals you've been eating.

How to Learn How Much Carbohydrate is in Your Food

There are several different ways to learn about how much carbohydrate is in your food. One is to pick up a book of nutritional information at your local library or bookstore, like those written by Corinne T. Netzer. Start browsing through it. Look up the foods you usually eat and see how many grams of carbohydrate are in a single portion. Though you can also find out how many grams are in a portion of food by Googling the food online, there are advantages to using a book. That's because books allow you to leaf through their pages and scan the nutritional information they contain quickly. Browsing through a book may also allow you to discover many foods with a low carbohydrate content that you might not have thought of looking up.

In all nutritional references, the carbohydrate content of foods is always given in grams. There are 28.3 grams in an ounce.

You can also look up nutritional information in apps like MyFitnessPal, on web sites like Fitday.com and calorieking.com, or on the USDA food database web site you will find online at: http://ndb.nal.usda.gov/ndb/foods.

Portion Size Matters

When you look up the carbohydrate count of a food, you must pay attention to the portion size to which that count applies. If your favorite muffin weighs six ounces, don't kid yourself that it has only 22 grams of carbohydrate. Yes, that may be the carbohydrate count you see listed in your nutritional guide for the entry, "blueberry muffin," but the portion size for muffins given in nutritional guides is almost always two ounces. Those huge muffins you find at your local coffee shop may weigh up to eight ounces each and may contain between 60 and 100 grams of carbohydrate.

You can also learn a lot about the carbohydrates in your food by reading the nutritional panels you'll find on boxed and canned foods. Again, note the portion size. Have you ever gotten 2.5 servings out of a can of Campbell's Soup? Me neither, but that's the portion size listed on the can.

An electronic food scale can be very helpful. Buy one and weigh the foods you eat at home for a few weeks until you get the hang of estimating portion size. Where the nutritional label printed on a processed food gives you both a weight and a measurement like "one half cup," the weight is always more accurate than the volume measurement.

An inexpensive food scale may be the best nutritional investment you'll ever make. When you weigh a serving of ice cream on a food scale, you'll quickly see that the "one serving" listed on the package turns out to be only a few tablespoons' worth. That bowl you've been considering as one portion of ice cream weighs in at four servings and turns out to provide 72 grams of carbohydrate and 600 calories. That may explain its damaging effect on both your blood sugar and your waistline.

Now that you know more about the foods that raised your blood sugar, it's time to see how much you can lower those post-meal blood sugar spikes just by lowering the amount of carbohydrate in your meals.

There are two ways of doing this. You can plunge right in or edge in gradually. We'll explain how to do both.

Safety Considerations when You Are Using Insulin, Drugs that Increase Insulin Production, or an SGLT2 Inhibitor Drug

Plunging right in can lower blood sugars dramatically. But if you are currently injecting insulin or if you are taking an oral drug that forces your beta cells to produce insulin, lowering carbohydrates dramatically is not a safe technique for you.

When you cut carbs, you produce less glucose, but if you are using a dose of insulin or an insulin stimulating drug that was designed for a high carbohydrate intake, you can easily suffer a dangerous low blood sugar hypo. So if you are using any of these drugs you'll need to proceed cautiously and talk to your doctor about how to reduce the doses of these medications as you reduce your carb intake. Remember, too, that it can take a few days for changes in your insulin or pill dose to take effect.

That is why, when you are using insulin or a drug that causes your beta cells to produce insulin, you must use the second technique described below, "Inching in slowly." With that approach, you can lower your medication gradually.

The oral drugs that stimulate insulin production are the drugs in the sulfonylurea family. They include glipizide (brand name: Glucotrol), Glyburide (Micronase, DiaBeta, Glynase), Gliclazide (Diamicron, Glizid, Glyloc and Reclide) and Glimepiride (Amaryl). Two other drugs that behave in a similar manner are Starlix (nateglinide) and Prandin (repaglinide).

The new family of SGLT2 drugs, which include Invokana, Forxiga, and Jardiance, can also make it dangerous to lower your carbohydrate intake to a level that is safe for people taking all other diabetes drugs. This is because they change the way that your kidneys function in a manner that can allow ketones to build up to dangerous levels in your bloodstream even when your blood sugars are normal. Ketone levels will start rising if your daily carbohydrate intake drops below a specific threshold that varies from person to person. Keeping your carbohydrate intake over 110 grams a day should keep most people above that threshold.

We will discuss these drugs further in Chapter Nine. But for now, if you are taking Invokana, Forxiga, Jardiance or any other drug in the SGLT2 inhibitor family, don't plunge right in, but use the "inching in slowly" technique described below, and make sure that you always keep your daily carbohydrate intake above 110 grams a day.

The other commonly prescribed diabetes drugs should not cause hypos or raise the risk of dangerous ketone levels when you cut back sharply on your carbohydrate intake. So if you are taking one of these, you can adopt either approach.

Modify Your Diet by Plunging Right In

The fastest way to lower your blood sugar is to remove all the carbohydrates from one of the meals you've previously tested and see what that meal does to your blood sugar when you eat it without any carbohydrates.

If you ate a burger, fries, and salad, for example, try eating only the burger without the bun and the salad. Instead of a sugary salad dressing such as raspberry vinaigrette, try oil and vinegar, Italian, blue cheese, or maybe ranch or parmesan peppercorn. All these are low in carbohydrate.

If a meal contains almost nothing but carbohydrates, for example, a breakfast of cereal, milk, and toast, try eating a different meal that contains the same amount of calories but has almost no carbohydrates such as eggs and ham without toast. Don't worry about fat content. If you are eating almost no carbohydrates, fats won't hurt you and they won't cause weight gain.

Test your no-carbohydrate or almost-no-carbohydrate meal one hour after eating and again two hours after eating, to see how the blood sugar spike that follows your reduced carbohydrate meal compares with the one you saw after eating the high carbohydrate version.

If you are like most people, you'll see a dramatic difference. Now remove as much carbohydrate as you can from the rest of the meals you tested earlier that raised your blood sugar over your chosen post-meal target. Keep doing this for at least two weeks. It takes a while for high blood sugars to drift down, but by the end of two weeks you should be seeing blood sugars that are much better than those you started out with.

As you lower the carbohydrate content of your meals, start adding portions of low carbohydrate vegetables to your diet, such as green beans, artichokes, asparagus, lettuce, spinach, brussels sprouts, broccoli, and cauliflower. Keep testing. These vegetables should not raise your blood sugars. If your blood sugars rise significantly after eating only the carbohydrates found in these very low carbohydrate vegetables, you may need to see an endocrinologist, as that would suggest you are making almost no insulin at all. You can also add low carbohydrate berries too. Raspberries, strawberries, and blueberries eaten in moderation should not raise your blood sugar.

Hunger

During the first two or three days after you've cut most of the carbohydrates out of your meals, you are likely to be very hungry. This is because your blood sugar will be dropping rapidly and your body is not used to that happening.

But if you can get through those two or three days your blood sugars will stabilize at a lower level and the hunger should disappear. What you should then experience is a new and delightful feeling of *freedom from hunger*. It is surprising how few days it takes for this to happen. So if you are hungry after eating your first few very low carbohydrate meals, tell yourself that the hunger is temporary, commit to sticking with the program for three days, and see how you feel when those three days are over.

If you want to snack, eat low carbohydrate snacks like cheese, sunflower seeds, meat, or one of the many low carbohydrate treats you can find online at low carb discussion boards or the Blood Sugar 101 web site.

Raising Your Carbohydrate Intake

Some people are extremely happy with how they feel while eating a very low carbohydrate diet. Others are not. It will take at least two weeks until you can evaluate the effect of a very low carbohydrate diet on your own, unique metabolism.

If you decide after a few weeks of eating a very low carbohydrate diet that this is not how you want to keep on eating, your next step should be to start testing your meals to see how much carbohydrate you can add back before your blood sugar rises back into the danger zone.

Try adding five more grams of carbohydrate to one of your very low carbohydrate lunches or dinners — breakfast can pose problems as most people, including those with completely normal blood sugars, are more insulin resistant at breakfast time. Test one and two hours after you eat that meal and see what happens. If you are still well below your chosen blood sugar target, add an additional five grams of carbohydrate to your next meal. Continue adding carbohydrate until you discover the amount of carbohydrate that pushes your blood sugar over your chosen blood sugar target.

Once you determine what amount of carbohydrates you can tolerate while still achieving your blood sugar targets you won't have to test every meal. Figure out how many grams of carbohydrate there are in the meals that work for you, and limit yourself to meals that contain that amount.

If it turns out that the maximum carbohydrate level you can tolerate is very low, don't panic. A well-chosen diabetes medication may allow you to raise your carbohydrate intake to where it is tolerable.

Modify Your Diet by Inching in Slowly

The other approach many people find helpful for getting back their blood sugar control is the inverse of the technique we just described. Here you take a meal that raised your blood sugar too high for safety and start whittling away at the carbohydrates it.contains a little bit at a time. This is the technique to use if you are using insulin or taking insulin-stimulating drugs or an SGLT2 inhibitor drug.

If your original meal was a hamburger, fries, and a salad, try the same meal without a bun. Test your blood sugar one and two hours after you finish eating, log your results, and see how much of an improvement you made by losing the bun. If you are seeing blood sugars higher than your target, try cutting out half the fries. Test again. If you are still over your target, eliminate the rest of the fries, or swap your sugary salad dressing and croutons for a low carbohydrate dressing.

If your breakfast of cereal and milk isn't working, try replacing the cereal with steel cut oatmeal. If that doesn't help, try a low carbohydrate flax cereal. Still too high? Try using almond milk instead of low fat or regular milk. If you still can't get a good reading, you'll have to take cereal off the menu. Try eating a low carbohydrate breakfast like eggs and meat instead.

Work through all the meals you enjoy, replacing the ingredients that raise your blood sugar too high with ones that are kinder. With this technique you can eat whatever you want—as long as you can reach the blood sugar targets you have set for yourself.

Undo the Damage Done by High Blood Sugars

As you read earlier, if you have been running very high blood sugars for many weeks or months, long-term exposure to these high blood sugars will have greatly increased the strength of your insulin resistance by adding secondary insulin resistance to whatever insulin resistance you were born with. This secondary insulin resistance makes whatever insulin your beta cells can make much less effective.

The great news is that, as you lower your post-meal blood sugars, you can eliminate this kind of secondary insulin resistance. If you achieve any of the blood sugar targets you saw in Table 4, after a few days your insulin resistance will start to decrease. Then whatever insulin you are still making will work more effectively, so that even without growing a single new beta cell, you will get a lower rise in blood sugar from each gram of carbohydrate you eat.

Even better, as your insulin resistance decreases, your liver may also become less insulin resistant and stop dumping loads of unneeded glucose into your bloodstream after meals. This, too, will bring your blood sugars down dramatically.

What Can You Achieve?

Surprisingly, how high your blood sugar is when you start this program does not predict how fast your blood sugars will drop or how many grams of carbohydrate you will end up being able to eat safely. I have seen people who started with extremely high blood sugars—ones far higher than mine—eat twice the amount of carbohydrate I can eat and still end up with blood sugars better than any I have ever been able to attain.

Your size and gender have a lot to do with it. The larger you are, the more carbohydrate your body can handle. Men typically can handle a bit more than women, even women of the same weight, possibly because they tend to have more muscle mass and muscle is what burns off most of our glucose.

The other factor that determines how far and fast you can progress is the degree to which your diabetes is caused by irreversible beta cell loss or dysfunction. If you have enough functional beta cells left, lowering insulin resistance will make a huge difference in your blood sugars. On the other hand, if your beta cells don't secrete insulin properly, or if your beta cells are dead, the amount of carbohydrate you can cover with the insulin you still make will be very limited.

There is no way to know if your high blood sugars are mainly caused by insulin resistance, insulin insufficiency, or a mixture of the two until you start lowering your carbohydrate intake and see what happens. For many people with Type 2 diabetes, what will happen is a very pleasant surprise. They achieve blood sugar numbers far better than what their doctor told them would be possible and do it without any need for medication.

For these lucky people, lowering their carbohydrate intake is all they need to do to normalize their blood sugar. For others it will be the first step, but other steps will have to follow. But it *is* the first step, so get yourself a meter and start testing!

Don't Be Fooled by False Hypos

As your blood sugar starts dropping toward the normal range, you may start experiencing low blood sugar symptoms. You may feel shaky or panicky a few hours after eating. At that point, you may fear you are heading for a dangerous low blood sugar attack and be tempted to eat some carbohydrates to raise your blood sugar back up.

Don't jump to the conclusion you are having a low blood sugar attack! Test your blood sugar. If it is over 70 mg/dl, [85 if you are using insulin or insulin stimulating drugs] reassure yourself that what you are experiencing is **normal blood sugar**. *If you are not injecting insulin* *or taking an insulin stimulating drug you do* not *have to worry about hypos!*

The word "hypo" is short for "hypoglycemia," which in turn is mangled medical-Greek for "low sugar." A true hypo is an emergency that occurs when too much insulin in your bloodstream causes your blood sugar drop so low that your brain can't function.

But if you are not using insulin or insulin stimulating drugs you shouldn't have to worry about dangerous hypos. Serious hypos aren't a problem for most people who are controlling their blood sugar using diet alone.

What you *are* likely to encounter as you lower your blood sugar is a **false hypo**. The false hypo makes you feel as if you are having a severe attack of low blood sugar when you aren't. And while it is uncomfortable, it is not a crisis. It is, in fact, a well-understood phenomenon that can happen if your fasting blood sugar has been elevated above truly normal levels for any period of time.

To understand the difference between a real hypo and a false hypo, you need to understand that a truly normal fasting blood sugar may range from 70 mg/dl up to the low 90s. That blood sugars as low as 70 mg/dl are safe is shown by the fact that doctors recommend that pregnant women keep their fasting blood sugars between 60 mg/dl and 90 mg/dl. This should make it clear that a blood sugar in the 60-70 mg/dl range is not a life-threatening emergency.

Hypos only become dangerous when blood sugar starts to drop into the 50s or lower. If your blood sugar drops into the 20s or 30s for an extended period of time you can become unconscious. This kind of hypo is a huge problem for people who inject too much insulin or take too much of an insulin-stimulating drug. But the only time a truly dangerous hypo will happen to a person who is not injecting insulin or taking an insulin-stimulating drug is if they have a rare endocrine disorder.

The reason you don't have to fear a hypo if you are not artificially raising your insulin level is that your body has an exquisitely sensitive feedback system whose job is to push your blood sugar back up as soon as it has dropped to more than 20 or 30 mg/dl below your usual fasting blood sugar level. When this happens, this system kicks in with dramatic effect.

It does this by secreting "counter-regulatory hormones" which are your old friends the "fight or flight" stress hormones. One good burst of counter-regulatory hormone and your blood sugar will surge back into the safe zone. Unfortunately, that burst of counter-regulatory hormone will also set your pulse pounding, your sweat glands pouring, and your body feeling as if you'd just narrowly escaped becoming a predator's lunch.

What makes the counter-regulatory response so hard to deal with for Type 2s—and what adds to the confusion about the danger of hypos—is that the body does not have a set, *absolute* threshold for responding to perceived hypos. It does not say to itself, "Uh-oh, blood sugar approaching 55, time to do Hypo Repair!"

Instead, it uses a *relative* threshold based on the fasting blood sugar level it is accustomed to. If you've been running a fasting blood sugar of 180 mg/dl and cut back on your carbohydrates for a few days, when your blood sugar drifts down to 120 mg/dl, your body may scream, "Blood sugar 60 mg/dl below normal! Hypo! Hypo!" even though your blood sugar is barely approaching a normal level.

When your heart is pounding and you are feeling shaky and faint, it is very tough to do nothing, especially since your brain is likely to be sending out signals to the effect that all would be well if you'd just scarf down some nice high carbohydrate food to "fix" the problem.

Don't!

Instead, when you feel hypo, grab your blood sugar meter and test. Unless your blood sugar is under 70 mg/dl don't do anything. [85 if you are injecting insulin or taking an insulin-stimulating drug.] It's not unusual to experience the symptoms of a false hypo, test, and discover that your blood sugar is actually *higher* than your usual fasting level.

The reason this happens is that, by the time you feel the impact of those stress hormones, they may have already forced your liver to dump a load of glucose into your bloodstream to raise your blood sugar. These stress hormones not only leave you feeling jangled, sometimes for hours, they may make you even more insulin resistant than usual for the next couple hours.

This false hypo response can be a major barrier on the road to achieving normal blood sugars. If you aren't prepared for it, you may end up sabotaging yourself by reacting to the symptoms of a false hypo by gobbling carbohydrates in the belief that you are fighting a life threatening hypo.

The best way to deal with a false hypo problem is to know that your body will reset its glucose "thermostat" over time. If you don't treat a false hypo as if it were an emergency, your body will eventually get used to a new, lower, fasting blood sugar. Then it will only give hypo signals when you are having a true hypo—which, if you are a Type 2 who is not using insulin or insulin-stimulating medications, will never happen.

When these adjustments are complete, and your body gets used to living with normal blood sugars, you'll feel far better than you did in the past when your blood sugar was high. The only "problem" you may then encounter is that if you eat the way you used to, the very high blood sugar levels you used to feel comfortable at will now feel horribly toxic. This is actually good, because that unpleasant feeling many of us experience when our blood sugars rise into the danger zone will motivate you to avoid eating the foods that cause those damaging highs.

Others Ways of Lowering Blood Sugar without Drugs

After the first edition of this book was published, I began to get a lot of inquiries from readers who had read in the media or seen doctors on TV promoting diets or surgical approaches they claimed "reversed" diabetes. The term "reversal" is a weasel word that doctors use in place of "cure" since using the word cure could get them sued or struck off as charlatans. But the average person assumes that reversal means cure, and who wouldn't prefer a cure to a lifetime of having to always watch what they eat, which is what you will have to do if you follow the approach we outlined above.

So lets take a closer look at these claims that diabetes can be "reversed" and see what the real facts are.

The Extreme Diabetes Diet Your Doctor May Prefer

The "test, test, test" approach we've described above is simple to explain, easy to understand, and relatively easy to follow. It lets you eat the foods you are used to eating and gives you a lot of freedom to decide which of those foods you will eat. You would think that this would recommend it to doctors, but that is far from the case. That's because most doctors and nutritionists have been heavily influenced by many decades of badly designed, poorly interpreted research that appeared to prove that eating fat causes heart disease.

Even though that advice has been completely refuted by now, both by careful reanalysis of the original research and by new research, doctors still hesitate to recommend any diet that allows people with diabetes to eat fat. Not only that, but doctors have also been told for decades that eating protein damages the kidneys of people with diabetes, though that, too, has been refuted by more up-to-date scientific work.

But because of these lingering prejudices, doctors will go to great lengths to avoid telling people with diabetes to eat a diet that cuts carbohydrates, because when carbs are cut to any significant extent, the calories they represent must be replaced by either fat—which is actually the healthiest approach—or extra protein.

This explains the popularity among doctors of what has to be the most extreme diet ever devised for people with diabetes, the Newcastle Diet. This was the invention of Dr. Roy Taylor, the English physician we met in the previous chapter bemoaning the fact that people with diabetes had no choice but to deteriorate. Some years later, Dr. Taylor found a way, he claimed, to change this situation and "reverse" his patients' diabetes entirely. He did this by feeding people newly diagnosed with Type 2 Diabetes a special, "balanced" diet where they ate only 600 calories a day for eight straight weeks.

This is a starvation diet, and because eating any diet that low in calories for more than a week can cause irreversible harm to your heart or a fatal imbalance of your body's electrolytes, this kind of extreme starvation diet can only be eaten under the watchful and well-paid eye of a physician. But Dr. Taylor claimed that after eight weeks of starvation, his patients had "reversed" their diabetes and recovered normal pancreatic function.

There is no real magic to this Newcastle diet. All Dr. Taylor really found was a way to prescribe a very low carbohydrate diet without raising the intake of fat and protein. A "balanced" 600 calorie diet will contain 200 calories from carbohydrate, which would be supplied by eating only 50 grams a day. And as you will quickly see if you try eating only 50 grams of carbohydrate a day for even a single week, eating that low an intake of carbohydrate will drop the blood sugars of almost anyone recently diagnosed with diabetes to normal levels—even when those 50 grams are combined with any amount of fat or protein.

So what Dr. Taylor was really doing was simply prescribing a very low carbohydrate diet, but taking out the fat and protein that make it possible to eat such a diet without suffering the physiological and psychological effects of a type of starvation that could be experienced outside of his clinic only by those imprisoned in concentration camps or third world prisons.

Dr. Taylor's research was published in 2011, and it is notable that no follow-up study has been presented to document that the "reversal" his diet supposedly achieved persisted after the subjects were declared cured. The only follow-up study he has published is one that found that his 8-week starvation diet was far less successful when given to a group of people who had been diabetic for more than eight years. Only half of those were able to achieve normal blood sugars with his extreme approach.

What we do know, however, is that there are many thousands of people who have been eating diets containing roughly those same 50 grams a day of carbohydrate, or quite a few more, accompanied by reasonable amounts of hunger-satisfying fat and muscle-preserving protein, who have maintained their normal blood sugars for years and even decades. Unlike Dr. Taylor's starvation diet, their diet lets them eat all the fat and protein they need to avoid being hungry, so it is sustainable, and requires no medical supervision to keep it safe. So why not make things easy on yourself, and follow the moderate path they have taken?

The Vegan Diabetes Diet—Much Hype, No Substance

Another diet for which there are claims that it "reverses" diabetes is the vegan diet. You will, however, only hear these claims from people who do not themselves have diabetes and who have not actually tried to reverse diabetes eating a vegan diet. This is due to the efforts of Dr. Neal Barnard a prolific author on health issues who has presented himself to the media as an expert in the treatment of diabetes. He is not. Though he is entitled to use the initials "M.D." after his name, Dr. Barnard was not trained in a medical specialty that would have allowed him to gain experience treating people with diabetes. *The New York Times* reported that he is a "nonpracticing psychiatrist."

Since completing his residency, what Dr Barnard has actually put his energy into doing is founding and leading a political group, deceptively named "The Physicians Committee for Responsible Medicine" (PCRM). PCRM is an extreme animal rights group whose sole aim is to force the public to stop eating animal products of any kind. *Newsweek* reported that only 5% of this organization's members are physicians. The rest of the membership includes laypeople, some of whom are members of radical animal rights groups that promote the use of violent tactics. Much of PCRM's funding comes from the extreme animal rights group, PETA.

Over the years, PCRM has worked tirelessly to frighten the general public about the dangers of the low carb dietary approach, since low carb dieters replace carbohydrates with the eggs, dairy, and meat that are anathema to vegan political campaigners. PCRM has used some very questionable methods to make its points, including nuisance lawsuits and, in at least one high-profile case, stealing and publicly releasing private medical records.

The sole medical study that Dr. Barnard has been involved with that in any way involves diabetes is a study that compared the old American Diabetes Association Diet—a very low fat, high carbohydrate diet—with a low fat, extremely high carbohydrate vegan diet. That study lasted over a period of 22 weeks with follow-up at 74 weeks—or approximately a year and a half. Several papers were published from this one study, and though Dr. Barnard's name appears on the papers, he does not appear to have been involved with conducting the actual research.

All participants in this study started out with A1cs averaging 8%. The group eating the vegan diet lowered their A1c on average by .96%--i.e. from 8% to 7.04%. This was .46% better than the A1cs of the people eating the ADA diet. But by 74 weeks, those eating the vegan diet had regressed. Their A1cs now were only lower than where they started by an average of .34%--i.e. their average A1c had dropped from 8% to 7.77%. The high carb ADA diet performed even worse, allowing Dr. Barnard to claim superiority for his diet.

Dr. Barnard's research was published at a time when many doctors and nutritionists were desperate to find some proof that the very low fat/high carbohydrate diet they had been promoting for years was not another failed fad diet. So the medical establishment welcomed Dr. Barnard's research, and the handsome, though completely unqualified, doctor was put onto committees that judged who should receive research grants and was even invited to star in three PBS health documentaries.

I will leave it to you to decide if a diet that requires you to give up most of the foods you are used to eating and replace all animal protein with vegetable proteins, especially that of the thyroid-poisoning soybean, is worth adopting just to achieve a decrease in A1c of .34%. But since Dr. Barnard's own research makes it crystal clear that his vegan diet leaves those who adopt it with A1cs closer to 8.0% than 7.0%, it is blatantly obviously that it has in no way been proven to "reverse" diabetes or even bring blood sugars down to a level that will prevent serious diabetic complications.

Over the many years I have maintained the Blood Sugar 101 web site I have heard from quite a few people with diabetes. I have occasionally heard from people who have improved their health eating the low fat ADA diet. I have even heard from someone who participated in Dr. Taylor's Newcastle diet trial and said that it did bring his blood sugars down to normal, though getting through that eight weeks of starvation was the toughest thing he had ever done. But I have yet to hear from anyone who normalized a diabetic blood sugar by eating an exclusively vegan diet. Perhaps they are out there, but if so, they are an oddly quiet group.

Weight Loss Surgery: A Dangerous Involuntary Low Carb Diet

The last approach your doctor—and more recently, your health insurer—may promote as being better than all these dietary approaches for "reversing" diabetes is weight loss surgery. The media are full of reports claiming that weight loss surgery can cure diabetes. So it should be no surprise that health insurers, increasingly overburdened by the expense of covering the high cost of the many patented diabetes drugs, are being heavily lobbied by surgeons' groups claiming that a single surgery—admittedly a very costly one—will eliminate the need to pay for years' worth of diabetes drugs.

There is no question that weight loss surgery can lower blood sugar. But though the surgeons who profit from this surgery like to suggest that this is because the surgery somehow alters physiology in some mysterious way that gets rid of the root cause of diabetes, the facts do not support this claim. Instead, as was the case with the Newcastle diet, the reason that these surgeries may appear to "reverse" diabetes is that they make it impossible for people to eat enough carbohydrates to raise their blood sugar out of the normal range.

After having weight loss surgery, people can only eat a few teaspoons full of food at a single meal, and many experience "dumping syndrome" — projectile vomiting — if they eat more than a tiny amount of carbohydrate at one time. Since it is carbohydrates that raise blood sugar, surgeries that make it impossible to eat carbohydrates will indeed lower blood sugar.

But this is a risky surgery — in the United States about 180 people a year die from it. So is it worth the risk? To answer that we have to look at the data that tracks how well this "diabetes cure" holds up over time. And that data is sobering.

A study published in the high impact journal, *Annals of Surgery*, in 2013 followed 217 people with Type 2 Diabetes who had had weight loss surgery over a period lasting between 5 and 9 years. One hundred and sixty-two had the radical Roux-en-Y gastric bypass operation, which irreversibly reroutes the path of food through the stomach and small intestine. Thirty-two had the potentially reversible gastric banding procedure where a band limits the size of the stomach, and 23 had the irreversible amputation of part of the stomach known as sleeve gastrectomy.

The study classified a subject as having experienced a "complete remission" — i.e. a cure — if they ended up with an A1c below 6.0% and a fasting blood glucose under 100 mg/dl while taking no diabetes medications. Five to nine years after surgery, 24% of those who had these surgeries experienced "complete remission." This, of course, implies that the remaining 76% still had abnormal blood sugars.

Among these, 34% were described as having "improved." The study defined "improvement" as meaning that the subjects experienced a drop in A1c greater than 1%. However, since the starting A1cs of the subjects in this study ranged up to 8.5%, a person could be considered "improved" if their A1c six years after surgery was still 7.45%--a level corresponding to an average blood sugar of 162 mg/dl. That level is still high enough to cause all the classic diabetic complications and it correlates with a greatly increased risk of heart attack. But there is more: A full 16% of those who had these major surgeries — one out of 6 — experienced *no improvement at all* in their blood sugars.

Over Time Weight Loss Surgery "Cures" Deteriorate

Another finding of this study seems to answer the question of whether this surgery actually affects some underlying physiological cause of diabetes. A full 19% of the people whose blood sugars initially normalized after surgery saw their blood sugars rise back into the diabetic range over time. This happened more frequently in people who had had diabetes for a longer time and whose weight loss was not maintained.

This reinforces the idea that it was carbohydrate restriction rather than any other effect of surgical body modification that explained the initial improvement in their blood sugars. People who have had this surgery report in online discussion forums that over time their stomachs stretch out to where they are able to hold more food. It is at this point that many start regaining weight. It is likely that this is also when they go back to eating the larger amounts of carbohydrate that raise their blood sugar back to the diabetic range. Rerouting or removing their stomachs did not do anything to modify the underlying physiological causes of their diabetes.

Since many people with diabetes can achieve A1cs in the 5% range by limiting carbs without artificial aid, it is worth trying the "test, test, test" diet before you go under the knife. And if cutting the carbs doesn't give you normal blood sugars, it isn't likely that this kind of surgery will either.

Chapter Seven
Making Your Diet Work

Okay, you've been using your meter to check out your meals, and it's starting to hit you that yes, it is those carbohydrates that are raising your blood sugar. Even better, when you cut back on the carbohydrates your blood sugar starts to drop dramatically and you begin to experience blood sugars far better than any you have seen since your diagnosis. But if your previous experience with restricting carbohydrates was a weight loss diet that worked well for you until you crashed off it entirely and gained back all the weight you'd lost, you may be hesitant to embark on another course of dieting that requires that you commit to restricting your carbohydrate intake.

If so, join the crowd. Sticking to a diet is always a challenge. Doing it when there is no end in sight and no time when you will reach goal and be able to lay off the dieting is even harder. So unlike all the other authors who promote low carbohydrate diets, I am not going to tell you that you will feel so great on the diet that you will adhere to it for the rest of your life and never have any problems sticking to it.

Maybe you will. I know a few people who have. But after years of reading the messages posted daily on the low carbohydrate diet newsgroup and even more years reading the diabetes discussion forums, my guess is that like most people who adopt long-term low carbohydrate diets you *will* run into problems—the same problems that derail most people who adopt these diets. So what I'm going to tell you now is that you should *expect* these problems and design a way of eating that incorporates the strategies known to solve them.

Weight Loss Diets Fail but Diabetes Diets Can't Afford To

Despite the alluring promises made by authors of bestselling diet books, most people who eat low carbohydrate diet to lose weight fail. They start out with great enthusiasm and during the early period when they are losing weight they swear they will never again eat another french fry or piece of toast. Some stick to their diets for months or even years. But after denying themselves so many of the foods everyone else around them is eating, most eventually burn out and slink back to their old eating patterns, usually gaining back all the weight they lost and more.

This is not a surprise. People on *any* diet—including a low calorie or low fat diet—do the same thing. The body is very resistant to weight loss. Instincts buried deeply in our brains do everything they can to raise our weight back to where it used to be, no matter how unhealthy that weight might have been. But while a failed diet may be tolerable for those who are dieting to shed a few pounds before their class reunion, it spells disaster when we must change our diet to prevent amputation, blindness, kidney failure, and heart attack.

Cutting carbs for diabetes means cutting them for life—long after the thrill has worn off of eating all that yummy cheese and steak. Despite the hype in the diet books, it is not easy, simple, and fun. After many years of participation in low carbohydrate diet support groups on the web, I have met only a handful of people who have been able to sustain a stringent ultra low carbohydrate lifestyle for more than five years. I sure couldn't.

But what I have observed over the same period of time is that there are a lot of people with diabetes who do the diet in a different way, and these people *have* been able to make a carbohydrate restricted diet work through years and even decades. They succeed because the approach they take is different in subtle ways from that of the weight loss dieter. Now let's look at how they do it.

The Tricks that Make a Life-Long Diabetes Diet Work

Focus on Your Blood Sugar Targets, Not Grams

When people think about adopting a lower carbohydrate diet, their first question is almost always, "How many grams of carbohydrates can I eat at each meal?" Most of the diet books will answer that question with a hard and fast number. Dr. Atkins, for example, tells you to start out with 20 grams a day. In *Protein Power,* Dr. Eades starts you at 30 grams. Dr. Bernstein suggests that you eat 6 grams for breakfast and snacks and 12 grams at lunch and dinner.

Adopting these very low carbohydrate limits will control your blood sugar very nicely. But over time, many people find that sticking to a diet this low in carbohydrate becomes impossible. That's why the approach we sketched out in Chapter Six did not tell you how many grams to eat. Instead all you have to do is eat the number of grams of carbohydrate that lets you meet the blood sugar targets you have set for yourself.

This is what The 5% Club calls **eating to your meter**. What you're doing when you eat to your meter is creating what Australian diabetes activist Alan Shanley calls *a low spike diet* rather than a low carbohydrate diet. Alan reports that he is able to keep his blood sugars under 140 mg/dl even when eating as many as 30 or 40 grams of carbohydrates at a single meal. Other people with diabetes find they must eat a lot fewer grams of carbohydrate than Alan eats to achieve safe post-meal blood sugar targets. But no matter how many grams they are eating, the result for all is the same: one hour post-meal blood sugars under 140 mg/dl.

In case you wonder, the reason why Alan can safely eat almost three times as many grams of carbohydrates without medications as I can is something that diet books rarely mention, though it is explained in detail in the book, *Dr. Bernstein's Diabetes Solution*. The explanation is that the amount of carbohydrate you can manage has a lot to do with your body size. The more you weigh, the less each gram of carbohydrate will raise your blood sugar. The same two grams of carbohydrate that will raise the blood sugar of a person who weighs 280 lbs only 5 mg/dl will raise the blood sugar of a person who weighs 140 lbs a full 10 mg/dl—twice as high.

In addition, as we saw earlier, while some of us are diabetic primarily because of high insulin resistance, others have high blood sugars because our beta cells have stopped secreting first or second-phase insulin, and yet others of us have trouble making basal insulin. The ease with which we can lower our blood sugar via diet alone has a lot to do with how much insulin we can still make and the extent to which the insulin resistance we experience is inborn rather than created by exposure to high blood sugars.

That is why testing your own carbohydrate tolerance is so essential. Through testing after meals you'll learn how many grams of carbohydrate your own, unique, body can handle. And more importantly, you'll also be able to decide if your body can handle enough grams of carbohydrate that it will be possible to control your blood sugar through a sustainable diet alone, or whether you will need to talk to your doctor about supplementing dietary control with drugs.

Take Care when Eating Away from Home

The biggest challenge you'll encounter as you change your diet to lower your blood sugar will be eating away from home. You aren't going to be able to weigh restaurant foods nor can you look up the nutritional values of many restaurant offerings. Even restaurants that provide nutritional guidance often provide counts based on much smaller portions than what they actually serve you.

This makes it a very good idea to avoid starchy or sugary restaurant foods or, if you do eat them, to eat only a small portion of what you are offered. Measure your blood sugar an hour or two hours after eating if you aren't sure about how a certain restaurant meal will affect you. Then the next time you visit that restaurant you'll have a better idea of what to order.

Avoid Becoming a Fanatic

Many people are so excited to learn that they can achieve normal blood sugars by cutting back on carbohydrates that they become zealots for low carbohydrate dieting. But it's important not to get too carried away with a "Carbs are Evil" mentality, which makes it a matter of religious dogma never to eat the evil carbohydrates you've sworn off of. Like all conversions, this one tends to fade out in time, and, when it does, backsliding will follow. You need to control your blood sugar for the rest of your life, not for just as long as your enthusiasm lasts. So don't make carbohydrate restriction a religion. Treat it as a strategy that, when used in combination with many other strategies, including medication and exercise, can give you normal blood sugars.

If you can be flexible and treat carbohydrate restriction as one of a variety of tools available to help you meet your blood sugar targets, you are more likely to maintain excellent blood sugars for years to come.

Eliminate "Habit Carbs" and Concentrate on "Value Carbs"

When you start testing your favorite foods, you are likely to find that many of them contain far more carbohydrate than your body can handle. Though this implies that, thanks to diabetes, you will never again be able to eat those favorite foods, the impact of this discovery is often blunted by the immense relief you feel when you discover that, despite your diagnosis, you can still achieve normal blood sugars. After all, most of us are happy to give up donuts if it means we can also give up worrying about amputations or blindness.

But after a few weeks of devotion to your new lower carbohydrate diet you are likely to find yourself dreaming about eating the cakes or muffins or french fries you've denied yourself. And as time goes on you may feel increasingly depressed about just how much of the food you love you can no longer eat.

Low carbohydrate enthusiasts will tell you that you shouldn't feel this way. Or they'll tell you that if you stick with the diet these feelings will go away. But I'm a person who stuck to a very low carbohydrate diet for over six years and I'd be the first to tell you that while that approach may work for some people, it won't for those of us who do not have a will of iron, a love of self-denial, and a natural preference for eating a diet made up mostly of fatty proteins and healthy vegetables.

Forbidding yourself a single bite of any carb-laden favorite food is a great way to program yourself for disaster. Fortunately, it turns out that most people with diabetes don't have to indulge in monk-like self-denial to get back their blood sugar control. Moderation can achieve a great deal, and though you *will* have to restrict carbohydrates, you can do this and still make room for some high carbohydrate foods that you have enjoyed all your life.

Why? Because a quick look at your daily carbohydrate intake will often reveal that the bulk of the carbohydrates you are eating are what I call "habit carbs." These are the carbohydrates you eat without a second thought because they are there. Not because they taste good. Not because you couldn't live without them. Just because over the years you've gotten into the habit of eating them every day.

Here is a list of some prime "habit carbs."

- ❖ Cafeteria mashed potatoes made from powder
- ❖ Limp french fries
- ❖ Squashy hamburger buns
- ❖ Cardboard toast
- ❖ Cold home fries
- ❖ Stale boxed cookies
- ❖ Tasteless cellophane-wrapped pastries
- ❖ Rancid potato chips
- ❖ Waxy chemical-laden candy bars
- ❖ Watery, artificially flavored "fruit" juice

How many of these flavorless, high carbohydrate foods have you been consuming every day just because they were there? Probably a lot more than you realize. For most of us, the high carbohydrate foods that are really delightful turn out to be few and far between. So before you lift that high carbohydrate forkful to your mouth, ask yourself, "Is this food thrilling me?" If not, put it down. If it is, eat it, but pay attention to the flavor. Is it as delicious as you expected it to be? Does it even have much flavor? Would a piece of nice cheese or a few low carbohydrate nuts be just as satisfying? The answers may surprise you!

Make a distinction between these "habit carbs" and what I call "value carbs," which are the carb-rich foods that really do deliver something worth indulging in from time to time. I'm not going to lie to you and tell you that you can eat them whenever you want. You can't. Not if you want to keep your blood sugar low enough to avoid developing diabetic complications. You aren't going to be able to eat them very often, and you may not be able to eat a normal portion of some. But by using the strategies described below, you should be able to eat enough of these foods to keep yourself from feeling deprived—and without derailing your diet or ruining your health.

Don't Create "Forbidden Fruits"

The key to long-term success is to avoid endowing any food with the power that comes from making it forbidden.

If you've avoided eating bread for a couple of months, that humble roll in the restaurant bread basket may call out to you with an irresistible siren song. If you give in and eat it, with each bite you may find yourself feeling as if you are doing something incredibly sinful—the way you might have felt if you had eaten a whole box of chocolates in the past—or committed adultery!

That feeling is the sign that you're heading for trouble. You've created a "forbidden fruit," and sooner or later that forbidden fruit is going to get you. You may declare that you will never again eat a roll—and then end up in tears your family's Thanksgiving dinner because you couldn't eat even a single one of Aunt Glenda's wonderful rolls that you have eaten at every Thanksgiving since you were small, the ones that say, "This is our family Thanksgiving."

You may start to dream of rolls night after night. You may find yourself craving rolls all day long, feeling that if you could only eat one roll you'd finally be happy. But of course diabetes has ruined your life, so you can't eat even one, which makes you totally depressed. Pretty soon you'll start resenting family members or co-workers who have the gall to eat rolls in your presence and finding yourself lecturing them about how they are poisoning themselves with each bite they take.

Once that happens, it is only a matter of time until you end up crashing off the diet. Friends and family will do all they can to "help" you stop eating a diet that is making you more grouchy and depressed by the day. And even if they don't, your common sense will kick in and tell you that no health benefit is worth being so miserable.

Then you will eat that roll and then another and another. The resulting feeling of being out of control will fill you with self-hatred, which will push you into old patterns of denial. You'll be relieved when your doctor assures you that an A1c of 7.4% is fine and that there is no reason to be more stringent. You'll stop participating in diabetes support groups where you might encounter information that challenges the denial you find so comfortable. You'll pack on weight and tell yourself you don't care.

Not a pretty picture? Eh? And not one sketched out in any of the bestselling diet books. But this is the scenario a lot of us have experienced after attempting to control our diabetes with carb-restricted diets that were far too stringent. That's why it is best to make room in your diet for a roll every now and then, to prevent it from building up a charge. When you give yourself permission to eat that object of desire every so often, you'll almost always find out that it doesn't taste anywhere near as good as you remembered. Then you'll be able to ignore that food for many more weeks without turning it into an object of obsession.

Knowing that you can eat those tempting off-plan foods at some future time when you have scheduled an off-plan meal will make it that much easier to say, "No thanks" to them the rest of the time. That approach makes it easier stick to a diet that does require that you mostly eat only those foods your body can handle.

Provide Safety Valves

This is why many people with diabetes find it helpful to build safety valves into our diets. We don't call them "cheats" or say we are "bad" when we eat them, because those terms carry an emotional burden that isn't helpful. We say we ate "off-plan" because we know these high carbohydrate foods are not foods we can make an ongoing part of our daily food plan because they *do* raise our blood sugars too high. These foods include indulgences like cake, pastry, bagels, and waffles.

Because our goal is life-long blood sugar control, we accept that most of the time we won't be able to eat these foods. If we do, we will harm our health. But we also accept that we are human, so we schedule occasional meals where we can eat "off-plan." We do this knowing that an occasional high blood sugar spike is not going to kill us as long as we are meeting our blood sugar targets the rest of the time. The "good enough" control we can adhere to year in and year out beats a few months of perfection followed by crashing off the diet entirely and ruining our health.

An occasional hour or two spent over those safe blood sugar targets won't harm you. It's when you spend two or three, or five, or six hours a day over your targets, day after day, that high blood sugars harm your organs. So if you go off-plan, let it be no more than one or two times a week. You are creating a safety valve for your food cravings, not a bad habit!

Do the Diet Straight Before You Try Off-Plan Goodies

Changing your diet is mostly a matter of changing your habits. To succeed at eating in a way that doesn't raise your blood sugar you will have to break a lot of established habits and replace them with new ones. So when you start out working on blood sugar control, it's a good idea to eat only the foods that keep your blood sugar in the safe zone for long enough to establish new and healthier habits. This usually takes a couple months.

Only when these new eating habits are firmly in place should you start working on the problem of how to deal with high carbohydrate temptations. Even so, knowing that you will be able to work some of those beloved foods back into your plan eventually should help you get through this break-in period.

For your first three months let your meter be your guide. If your meter tells you a food raises your blood sugar over your target level, don't eat it again. Eat only the foods your blood sugar can tolerate.

When you eat only the foods that don't raise your blood sugar, several things will happen. Within a few days you should stop feeling hungry. For the first time in years you may find yourself no longer dominated by food cravings and the relentless need to eat. The discovery that these cravings were not due to an emotional problem but were caused entirely by the high blood sugar spikes you were experiencing will be enormously reassuring. From then on, as long as you are controlling your blood sugar and getting enough calories to provide your metabolic needs, you shouldn't feel hungry. Remind yourself: *hunger is always a symptom.*

An interesting thing will happen after you cut a lot of sugar out of your diet. After a few weeks your sense of taste will change and you may be surprised to discover that vegetables taste much better than they used to. When you do eat something with sugar in it, you may find its sweetness almost unpleasant—far too sweet for your reeducated taste buds. These changes in your hunger level and sense of taste can make it easier to stick with a carb-restricted diet for a long time without feeling unduly deprived.

If you attempt to add off-plan foods before you are solidly on-plan, you may never really get to this point. Most people who crash on and off low carbohydrate diets do so because they don't eat at a carbohydrate intake level low enough to control their blood sugar for long enough to experience the benefits that would motivate them to continue.

When you have finally gotten your blood sugar under control and started to enjoy those benefits, nothing horrible will happen if you make room for some high carbohydrate treat every now and then. This may be heresy to some people committed to a low carbohydrate diet, but I am convinced that it is the best way to ensure that this year's enthusiastic carb-restricted dieter is still a happy 5% Club member ten, or twenty, or fifty years from now. And you do want to maintain your health for that long, don't you?

How Often Can You Eat Off-Plan?

How often you can eat an off-plan food depends a lot on your dietary goals, how well you tolerate carbohydrates, and whether you are willing to exercise after eating. It also depends greatly on what medications you are taking for your diabetes.

Forty minutes of running, biking, weight lifting, or even brisk walking will burn off some extra carbohydrate. So if you exercise regularly, try to eat your high carbohydrate treat before you head for the gym. Your meter will tell you if your exercise session burned off enough glucose to lower your blood sugar.

However, if you are also trying to lose weight, be careful! A lot of research suggests that most dieters greatly overestimate how many calories they burn through activity. The "calories burned" data provided by fitness trackers and gym machines are often much higher than those seen when exercisers' energy consumption is carefully measured in the lab. And because calories really do count, if you're trying to lose weight, you have to consider more than just your blood sugar level when considering what to eat.

Some people like to schedule their off-plan meal for a specific time—Saturday night, perhaps. Others decide to eat one or two off-plan meals every week at whatever times best suit their lifestyle. What you decide to do, of course, is up to you.

Indulge with Portions You Can Tolerate

When it is time to eat off-plan, it often helps to fill up with foods that are good to your blood sugar and then eat a small portion of the foods you find hard to handle.

If you are craving donuts, try eating one donut hole. Make a sandwich with one slice of bread not two. Eat one scoop of ice cream. Throw out half the fries before you eat the rest. Your goal is to eat enough to defuse its hold over you and, most importantly, to rediscover that few of these very high carb foods are anywhere near as good as you remembered them being.

Throw Away the Vocabulary of Self-Destructive Dieting

When you eat something with carbohydrates in it, don't think of it as a "cheat." Cheating is what you do when you're under the thumb of some authority figure—be it your 9th grade math teacher or the IRS. But *you* are the one in control of what you eat. So when you eat something that is off-plan, don't think of it as getting away with something. It is something you've decided to do for a very good reason.

Avoid getting into a power struggle with yourself. You'll always lose! If you keep eating things that you didn't mean to eat, rather than beating yourself up, take it as a sign that your current food plan isn't working. Then put some energy into figuring out *why* it isn't working.

Are you having trouble finding foods in restaurants that don't raise your blood sugar? Maybe it's time to bring a lunch to work for a while or to find a new place to dine. Are you bored with what you have been eating? Google the web for low carbohydrate recipes or join one of the big diabetes or low carb diet discussion boards on the web where hundreds of members exchange recipes and ideas for interesting things to eat.

At **lowcarbfriends.com** or **forum.lowcarber.com** you will find many people who have done well eating a long-term low carbohydrate diet and who are eager to help you succeed. Just be aware that these forums also have a certain number of active participants who are paid to plug expensive, low carb junk foods made out of bizarre lab-created ingredients, many of which contain more carbohydrate than their labels claim. Others will be touting expensive miracle supplements, whose claims we will discuss further in Chapter Eleven. Stick to the recipes you find online whose ingredients are real foods you can buy at your supermarket. They are more likely to be kind to your blood sugar.

Get Your Nutrient Balance Right

If you have been eating in a way that controls your blood sugar for more than a few weeks, but still find that your diet is making you hungry, try tweaking it. Are you eating too little food? Too little protein? Too much protein? Too little fat? Too much fat? Too few vegetables?

A healthy carb-restricted diabetes diet should not be a low fat diet. Nor should it be a high protein diet. Determining exactly how much fat you should eat requires understanding that the lower your carbohydrate intake is, the more fat you can eat safely.

If you are eating a very low carb **ketogenic diet**, which is defined as a diet that provides less than 70-100 grams of carbs a day, depending on your body size, which switches your muscles to burning fat rather than glucose, it is safe to eat up to 70% of your daily calories in the form of healthy fats, eating only as much protein as is needed to meets your nutritional requirements. The Atkins Diet is a ketogenic diet.

However, because decades ago the celebrity doctors promoting ketogenic diets labeled them "high protein" diets, rather than high fat diets, to cater to society's fat phobia, many people make the mistake of eating too much protein when they eat very low carb ketogenic diets. When eating a ketogenic diet it is much better, for many reasons, to replace most of the calories you cut when you eliminated carbohydrates with those from fat. Not the least of these reasons is that eating only as much protein as you really need will cure the bad breath that is so common among dieters eating very low carb ketogenic diets.

You can find out exactly how much protein and fat you should eat at any given carbohydrate intake level by using the Metabolic Calculator you will find on the Blood Sugar 101 web site at: **http://www.phlaunt.com/diabetes/DietMakeupCalc.php**.

How Much Fat Is Healthy Depends on Your Specific Carb Intake

Though it is safe to eat a very high amount of fat with a very low carb ketogenic diet, many people who are cutting back on carbohydrates to control their blood sugars aren't eating a ketogenic diet providing less than 100 grams of carbohydrates a day. Instead, they are eating a *moderate* carb-restricted diet. If that's your situation, you will want to ignore the many recipes and eating strategies that are labeled as being suitable for "low carb dieters." Those assume that the dieter is eating a ketogenic diet and provide the very high percentage of fat that is only healthy when people are eating ketogenic diets.

But the very high fat intake that is healthy for ketogenic dieters can be a problem for people eating more moderate carb-restricted diets, which includes many people with diabetes who cut carbs just enough to control their blood sugar in a way that is sustainable over a lifetime. Research has shown that the high fat intake that is healthy when a person is eating 80 grams a day of carbohydrate becomes unhealthy when their daily carbohydrate intake rises over 150 grams a day. One reason that there is so much older research showing that low carbohydrate diets are unhealthy is that until the early 2000s all "low carb" diet research was done with diets that provided 150 grams of carbohydrate a day along with a lot of fat, and those diets were indeed unhealthy.

By the time your carbohydrate intake has risen to where it is 40% of your daily calories, compelling diet research, discussed in depth in my book, *Diet 101: The Truth About Low Carb Diets*, has shown that the healthiest nutrient breakdown is that prescribed by the Zone Diet— 40% carbs, 30% fat, and 30% protein. At a 40% carbohydrate intake level, if fat intake rises higher than 30% blood lipids will deteriorate, as will other measures of metabolic health. Not only that, but a high fat intake with a moderate carbohydrate intake is a great way to gain weight.

So if you are eating more than 110 grams of carbs a day—a level that is no longer considered a very low carbohydrate diet level, stay away from the blue cheese dressing, cream sauces, and other very high fat foods that are appropriate only for people eating a very low carb diet.

Greens are Essential!

A long-term carb-restricted diet should also be one that is filled with leafy greens like romaine lettuce or kale and it should also include lots of the other low carbohydrate vegetables. Ideally, you should eat a big green salad every day and several other servings of low carb veggies like green beans, zucchini, or avocado. If you crave fruit, eat berries. If they are too expensive to buy fresh, buy them frozen and add them to one of the many low carbohydrate pancake recipes you can find online.

Eliminate the Chemical Additives that Make Us Hungry

Another thing that can make you hungry is over-use of artificial sweeteners. A growing body of research suggests that artificial sweeteners increase appetite in both rodents and people. Cut out the diet soda and drink herbal teas or seltzers for a few weeks to see if that helps.

MSG will make you hungry too. It occurs naturally in soy sauce and it is present in many packaged foods though you won't see it in the list of ingredients. Instead its presence is hidden by the use of alternative names like "hydrolyzed vegetable protein" or "natural flavoring."

If you have eliminated sweeteners and MSG and are still feeling hungry, perhaps you need to eat more fiber. Add a fiber cracker to each meal and see if that helps.

Whatever you do, keep the vocabulary of sin and guilt for the confessional. Your diet is not a moral issue, it's a metabolic one. Don't say, "I've been bad," say, "I went off-plan." You're going to eat a lot of things in the years to come that will mess up your blood sugar. When you stumble, be kind to yourself. Dust yourself off and keep on going. Blood sugar control is a marathon, not a sprint.

Go into this knowing you are going to slip up, and when you do, just recommit to doing the best you can. If you hit your chosen blood sugar targets more often than not, you will end up a lot better off than if you don't try. The important thing is to keep at it, doing the best you can, and to forgive yourself when the best you can do isn't as good as you wish it were.

Know Your Limits

I've learned the hard way I can't eat *half* a blueberry muffin, so I don't try to use portion control for that particular food. I know blueberry muffins are trouble and I also know that I will eventually eat one. That's just how it is. Every blue moon or so I eat a blueberry muffin, experience the miserable high blood sugars that follow, and then remember why I don't eat muffins every day. What I don't do is fool myself that I can buy a muffin and only eat half. Everyone has a few foods that fall into this category. Treat them with caution!

Eat Off-Plan Foods Out of the House

I've also learned that if a big box of something full of carbohydrates is in the fridge, bad things are going to happen. So I try to eat my off-plan foods away from home. I eat my muffins or cookies at a coffee shop. I have one slice of pizza at a pizzeria. I don't buy a box of muffins or a whole pizza and bring them home.

Getting this strategy to work requires that your whole family understand what's at stake. It took me a couple years of harping on what "complications" means, but by now my family understands that if my blood sugar is too high, I'm damaging my body. They want to keep me around for a while and agree that I'm cuter with all my toes. So they understand that there are some foods that shouldn't be brought into the house—ever.

When other family members want to have treats at home, they are kind enough to buy things I don't like. For example, if someone wants Ben & Jerry's they buy the Chunky Monkey flavor I find revolting not the New York Super Fudge Chunk.

Be Aware of Foods that Give Misleading Test Results

Some foods, including some often recommended for people with diabetes, give misleading test results. They may not cause spikes in the hours after you eat but still raise your blood sugar in a way that can make you hungry and stress your blood sugar control. We'll look at some of them here.

Carbohydrates Eaten with a Lot of Fat will Digest Slowly

Foods with a lot of fat in them take longer to digest than those without a lot of fat. This is why pizza and ice cream often give deceptively good readings on your meter. If you test a meal and see a reading at one and two hours after eating that is too good to be true, be sure you test at three or four hours after eating. If you notice yourself getting hungry several hours after eating certain meals that test well, it is possible that you are missing spikes occurring later than you expected.

The Truth About Pasta

Pasta was long recommended to people with diabetes as a food that would not raise blood sugar. This is why you will still see it starring in many "Diabetic" cookbooks and magazines.

Pasta made out of boxed dry noodles—not fresh pasta—usually doesn't raise blood sugar one hour after you eat and rarely after two. But if you test four or five hours after eating that pasta, you may get an unpleasant surprise. This is true even of the so-called "low carb" pastas. These pastas give you excellent readings at one and two hours because they are resistant to digestion, so they don't turn into glucose right away. But five hours later, they *do* digest into glucose and when they do, the 52 grams of carbohydrate found in each two ounce pasta serving may hit your bloodstream with a nasty wallop. Not to mention that you almost need a microscope to see a two ounce portion of pasta. Most people's idea of a portion of pasta is closer to six ounces—and 156 grams of carbohydrate!

If you have pasta for dinner and don't see a peak by two hours after you have eaten, be sure to check your fasting blood sugar the next morning. You may see an unexpected blood sugar rise then, which came from the pasta you ate the night before.

The people who can eat pasta or any kind of starch that resists digestion without seeing a spike hours later are those who still have a robust second-phase insulin release. If you find a food containing a resistant starch that appears to work well for you, and if you don't detect a delayed spike hours later, you can conclude you still have a significant second-phase insulin release left.

"Sugar Free" Foods Can Be Full of Carbohydrate

"Sugar free" foods are sold all over and promoted as being perfect for people with diabetes. The truth is that while they may not contain sucrose—table sugar—they are full of carbohydrates. Sugar free brownies or cookies are full of starchy flour. Sugar free ice cream is full of chemicals deceptively called "sugar alcohols" which are very different from the kind of alcohol you drink. These sugar alcohols are lab-created carbohydrates that may or may not break down into glucose in your body depending on whether you have the enzymes needed to digest them. If you don't, they won't raise your blood sugar, but they may give you horrible gas and diarrhea, since there are bacteria in your gut that can ferment these otherwise indigestible sugars. If they don't give you the runs, they probably *will* raise your blood sugar because that means you can digest them. But because they digest slowly you may not see the blood sugar spike they cause when you test one or two hours after eating.

Again, as is the case with digestion-resistant starches, whether you can eat foods containing sugar alcohols without raising your blood sugar will have a lot to do with how much second-phase insulin release you have left.

Of all the sugar alcohols used in making "sugar free" products, maltitol is the one that is most likely to raise blood sugar. At least half of every gram of maltitol digests into glucose within three hours. So if a "sugar free" food seems to be kind to your blood sugar, try testing it an hour or two after you usually test. Erythritol is the one sugar alcohol that does not raise blood sugar, but it is rarely found in commercial "sugar free" products.

Fructose — the Great Deceiver

You may have heard that fructose is preferable to other sugars for people with diabetes because it doesn't raise blood sugar. This is true because only glucose raises blood sugar, which is also known as blood *glucose*. Fructose is a different simple sugar. Because it is found in fruits, it is often portrayed as being "natural" and "healthy." However the fructose you find listed in the ingredient panel of supermarket foods does not come from fruit. It is extracted from corn. And no matter what its source or how kind it is to blood sugar, no form of fructose is good for people with diabetes.

Though fructose doesn't raise your blood sugar, it makes a beeline for your liver where it is immediately turned into a kind of fat that increases insulin resistance. Not only that, but dietary fructose also appears to decrease leptin, a hormone that regulates appetite and body fat levels.

The reason humans are so drawn to fructose probably goes back to our evolutionary primate heritage. Fat is hard to come by for most primates as they don't eat much meat, but they need to store fat to survive periods of famine. So, since primates get so much of their body fat from the fructose in the fruits they consume, our primate brains appear hardwired to eat as much fructose as possible. This only becomes a problem when our human bodies encounter huge amounts of this "fruit" sugar every day while never encountering the famine. Since table sugar is made of sucrose, a molecule that is one half fructose and one half glucose, this may explain why we find it so seductive and why the health consequences of eating sugar, whose fructose gets turned into liver fat, may be worse than those of eating the same amount of starch.

American's average consumption of sugar rose from 64 grams per day in 1970 to 81 grams per day in 1997 — a rise of 26% — and that was just the *average* consumption. Drink one sweetened latte and a 20 ounce bottle of regular Pepsi and you're already at 110 grams!

Agave Syrup, which is sold as a "natural" "health food" is 90% pure fructose, which is far higher in fructose than high fructose corn syrup.

Carb Blockers

Drug stores and web sites offer "natural carb blockers" which contain a bean extract that the makers claim keep carbs from being digested. While there is a prescription drug that *is* effective in blocking the digestion of starches and complex sugars, these supposedly "natural" blockers do not appear to be very effective, so you won't see them recommended by regulars on online diabetes forums. If any supplement actually does block the digestion of starch or sugar, you will experience an increase in intestinal gas, as undigested starches are fermented by gut bacteria. If any "carb blocker" appears to work, test your blood sugar three or four hours after eating, as the "blocker" may only be slowing digestion.

Don't Confuse Gluten-Free with Low Carb

Back in the late 1990s, when I first started watching my blood sugar, going gluten-free was a very good way to control blood sugar, because eliminating gluten forced you to eliminate most high carb junk foods: cake, cookies, snack crackers, and the many packaged, processed foods that had wheat starches added as filler.

But the advent of the gluten-free diet fad has changed that. Supermarkets, bakeries and restaurants are now filled with a huge range of gluten-free foods, which are as high in carbohydrates as the foods they replace—or higher. While there may be some health benefits to eliminating gluten from your diet, carbs are carbs, and gluten-free carbs will raise your blood sugar just as high as any other carbs and do the same amount of damage to your body.

Select Truly Healthy Foods as You Change Your Diet

Most people find that meats, nuts, and cheeses don't raise their blood sugar, so they eat more of them when they start getting serious about lowering their blood sugar. This will work well, as long as you are careful to avoid the processed versions of these foods that are likely to contain added chemicals that, though they might not raise your blood sugar, can be dangerous to your overall health.

Avoid Foods with Hidden MSG

We mentioned earlier that Monosodium Glutamate (MSG) can make you hungry and that it is often added to meats and packaged foods disguised by legally permitted pseudonyms. But the problems with MSG go beyond their impact on your appetite.

Though eating a bit of MSG now and then won't hurt you, eating it frequently has been shown to promote weight gain independent of how many calories are eaten. People eating the identical diet with MSG added have been found to be three times as likely to be overweight as those eating the same diet without it.

Some of the legally permitted pseudonyms for MSG include: natural flavoring, textured protein, hydrolyzed protein, yeast extract, glutamate, glutamic acid, calcium caseinate, hydrolyzed corn gluten, monopotassium glutamate, sodium caseinate, yeast nutrient, yeast food, natrium glutamate, and autolyzed yeast.

Added Inorganic Phosphates Present Another Serious Threat

Inorganic phosphates are another kind of additive whose effects on health should be of particular concern to people with diabetes. That is because consuming an excess of these chemicals has been shown to damage the kidneys and promote the formation of plaques in the arteries, raising the risk of heart attack.

Though naturally occurring *organic* phosphates are essential to the functioning of every cell in our bodies, they are very different from the ground up rocks that make up the family of inorganic phosphates. These include calcium phosphate, disodium phosphate, calcium pyrophosphate, and quite a few other chemicals. Unlike the organic phosphates, these inorganic phosphates, are not very bioavailable. So the phosphate they contain tends to remain in circulation in the blood until it precipitates out either in the kidneys or the arteries.

Inorganic phosphates don't occur naturally in food. They are added to packaged, processed foods, as preservatives, flavor additives, and to keep liquids like milk or coconut milk from separating during storage. They are also added to brown sodas in a liquid form, phosphoric acid, which is converted to phosphate in our bodies. This phosphoric acid keeps brown sodas like Coke or Pepsi from turning an unappetizing black. Phosphates are also sometimes used to provide the chalky white material that binds vitamins and supplements you buy in pill form. They are also major component in the baking powder used in cakes, crackers, and cookies.

It has long been known that consuming inorganic phosphates can be very dangerous for people with severe kidney disease, as failing kidneys can't remove phosphates from the blood, and these phosphates precipitate out in the kidney, destroying what little function is left. But while doctors may be aware of this, few know that consuming inorganic phosphates also poses a major risk to *normal* people, because it can promote heart disease.

We know from several well-conducted studies that there is a direct link between serum phosphate level and heart disease. As a recently published review article explains,

> Higher serum phosphate levels were independently associated with coronary artery calcification, vascular stiffness, left ventricular hypertrophy, and carotid artery disease, even among individuals with normal kidney function and serum phosphate levels within the normal range.

The Framingham Offspring study also found that normal participants whose serum phosphate levels fell in the upper 25% of the range of readings for the whole research group at the beginning of the 16 year study had a 55% higher risk of developing cardiovascular disease by the end of the study. This is a big leap in risk, especially when it is attributed to a factor that is completely ignored by doctors, health authorities, and food companies.

What raises serum phosphate levels? Elegant research has established that they rise along with a rise in the intake of inorganic phosphates. Subjects who were fed two different diets that were nutritionally identical, save that one had inorganic phosphates added and the other didn't, experienced much higher serum phosphate levels when they were fed the diet with the added phosphates.

There is no requirement that labels list how much added inorganic phosphate is found in a given food, which makes it very hard to know if you are taking in more than the recommended daily inorganic phosphate dose of 1 mg. Measurements suggest most people eating processed foods are getting far more than that.

Phosphates are a particular concern to people lowering their intake of carbohydrates because they are added to many convenience foods that would otherwise be very appealing, for example, they are found in most rotisserie chickens, half and half and cream, processed cheeses, and many packaged dinners sold in stores that cater to people who want "health food."

Read labels and do what you can to keep your intake of inorganic phosphates as low as possible. People with diabetes already have enough threats to their kidneys and arteries.

Dealing with Limited Blood Testing Supplies

In an ideal world, everyone would have all the testing supplies they need. But in real life blood sugar test strips are very expensive and many insurers sharply limit the number of strips people with Type 2 Diabetes can get each month.

Here are some strategies that can help you if your access to strips is limited:

❖ If you only have a limited number of strips to get you through a month, use them to learn when your highest blood sugar is likely to occur after a meal. Do this by testing several meals one hour, one and a half hours, and two hours after eating. People who still have a significant second-phase insulin release will usually see a peak one hour after the end of their meals. Others may see a later peak. Once you know the time when you are likely peak, test only at that time except when eating foods that are likely to be delayed, like pasta or foods with sugar alcohols. Test those foods an hour or two later.

❖ Make the goal of your testing be to learn how many grams of carbohydrate you can tolerate in one meal. If you learn that 20 grams is your upper limit, use software and your food scale to find portions of other foods that will also clock in at 20 grams or less. Test one or two of these portions. If you see the result you expect, you don't have to test when you eat that same amount of carbohydrate again.

❖ If you need more strips, consider the $35 you pay for a cheap meter and another 50 strips an investment in your health. It's far better to spend that $35 now, than to spend it on expensive doctor bills caused by complications you don't need to develop.

Medications Can Help

I'm not a big fan of medications because there is just too much evidence that drug companies lie about side effects. I learned the hard way that some of these side effects are unpleasant and permanent. But I learned the hard way, too, that some of us—like, say, me—can't get normal blood sugars no matter how low our carbohydrate intake. For us, adding a diabetic drug or two to our daily regimen may be the only way we can get normal blood sugars.

Adding one of the safer drugs may also make it possible for us to raise our carbohydrate intake to a level that is easier to sustain. Even a slight increase in intake can make a big difference psychologically. If you've only been able to hit your blood sugar targets by limiting yourself to eating 60 grams of carbohydrate a day, the 120 grams a day you can manage with the help of a safe diabetes drug is likely to feel like a completely normal diet.

We'll discuss the various drugs that may help you control your blood sugar in the next two chapters. Just remember that all the safe diabetes drugs work best when combined with some level of carbohydrate restriction. How much restriction? After you've started a new medication, test your meals one and two hours after eating, and your blood sugar meter will tell you exactly how much carbohydrate you can eat with your new medication while still hitting your blood sugar targets.

Chapter Eight
Generic Diabetes Drugs

Though many people diagnosed with Type 2 Diabetes find that they can bring their blood sugar back into the normal range simply by limiting their carbohydrate intake, not everyone is willing or able to stick with a restrictive diet for the rest of their lives. That's why most doctors assume that dietary changes will not solve their patient's blood sugar problems and prescribe **oral antidiabetic drugs** almost immediately after diagnosis. If these pills don't lower the patient's A1c to 7.5%, they may add one of the drugs like Victoza, Bydureon, or Trulicity, which, though they are injected, are not insulin.

Though they are called "antidiabetics" some of these drugs are occasionally prescribed for people whose blood sugars are prediabetic, since large studies have shown them to be effective for people with impaired glucose tolerance. You may well be asking, if these drugs are so effective, why should you bother with a complex and restrictive dietary regimen?

Effective, But Not Effective Enough

The catch is how you define "effective." Just as the American Diabetes Association's suggested blood sugar targets ignore the evidence pointing to the blood sugar levels at which organ damage occurs, the standard used by the FDA when it approves a drug as "effective for lowering blood sugar" falls well short of requiring that the drug bring blood sugar levels down to a level low enough to prevent complications.

So while an oral antidiabetic drug might be considered "effective" by the FDA, this only means that the drug lowers the blood sugar of a person with a very high blood sugar slightly better than does taking no drug at all. A drug that lowers an A1c of 10% to 9.5% is considered effective, even though the person taking it ends up with an average blood sugar of 261 mg/dl—a level high enough to guarantee complications.

When drugs are approved for use by people whose blood sugars are in the prediabetic range, they only need to lower an OGTT result by 20 or 30 mg/dl to be considered effective. Since many people diagnosed with prediabetes have blood sugars that go up to 180 or 190 mg/dl after each meal, these drugs could still leave a prediabetic person with blood sugars that are well above 140 mg/dl for most of the day.

The limited power of these drugs to lower blood sugar is why oral antidiabetic drugs, whether taken alone or in combination with non-insulin injected drugs, are not likely to bring your blood sugars back into the normal range. They are an add-on — not a substitute — for dietary control. But here's the silver lining: if you restrict your carbohydrates and are still unable to get your blood sugars back into the normal range, the addition of a well-chosen oral antidiabetic drug *may* push your blood sugar down that last little bit you need to normalize them.

Since I wrote the last edition of this book, a large number of new drugs have come onto the market. Many are copycat drugs, which are very similar in how they work to existing drugs. Doctors often switch patients to these new drugs even when they don't lower blood sugar any better than older drugs, including those in the same drug family. Sometimes they prescribe new drugs that do a *worse* job of lowering blood sugar than existing drugs. This is because new drugs are released with huge marketing budgets and aggressive sales campaigns that make exaggerated claims about their health benefits. These claims rarely hold up to the test of time, but it takes years for impartial academic research to disprove them. In the meantime the companies promoting these new drugs earn billions.

The side effects of new drugs are also unknown, making them attractive to doctors who are all too aware of the side effects of the older drugs they have been prescribing. Most of the clinical trials required for drug approval only involve a few hundred or thousand patients who take the drug for a few years. But it is only after hundreds of thousands of patients use a new drug for a decade or more that some of the most severe side effects become evident.

Even worse, when evidence of these severe side effects does emerge, the big drug companies have a long and ugly history of suppressing the publication of the studies that uncover it or of bribing doctors to keep prescribing them. So you will often have to wait until a drug's patent has expired to learn what its real side effects have been. By then hundreds of thousands of people will have taken the drug and many will have suffered these side effects.

With that in mind, next we will take a closer look at the drugs your doctor is most likely to prescribe for you and examine what research has found about what they do well, what they do poorly, and what you need to know before deciding whether any particular drug might be worth trying.

In this chapter we will discuss the diabetes drugs that have been on the market long enough to have lost patent protection so that they are now available in generic forms. We'll cover the newer, brand name drugs in the next chapter.

There are good reasons to consider some of these generic drugs. One is that because they *are* generic these are the drugs health insurers will usually put in the tier with the cheapest copay. But a more important reason to consider these drugs first is that because they have been on the market for so long we have had enough time to learn the facts about what they really do and what their real side effects are.

Unfortunately, because these drugs are now cheap, the salespeople who visit doctors no longer remind them of these drugs' capabilities, while they are continually hammering home the dubious benefits of the newer, expensive, patented drugs that we will be discussing in the next chapter. So doctors often are swayed to prescribe the newer drugs to any patient whose insurance will pay for them, even though, as you will see, several of the older, generic drugs may be superior.

So with that in mind lets start by looking at the diabetes drug with the longest history and the best record for safety and efficacy.

Metformin

Metformin was first discovered in the late 1950s. It has been used to control diabetic blood sugars in Europe since the 1970s and in the United States since the mid 1990s. It's now available in very cheap generic versions, so drug reps no longer push it except when it is combined with a newly released drug in a single expensive pill. But unlike the new drugs, metformin has a long safety record and has been the subject of many studies, some tracking its impact for decades— something no drug still under patent can claim. This means we have a very good idea of what its real benefits and side effects are.

Ongoing research has revealed that many of metformin's side effects are beneficial, unlike those of all the other oral diabetes drugs we'll be discussing. Several studies published since 2010 document quite convincingly that metformin, alone among the diabetes drugs, has "side effects" that include a dramatically lower risk of death from heart disease and a possible anti-cancer effect. In addition, metformin also helps make weight loss easier.

The current American Diabetes Association practice recommendations state that metformin should be the first drug prescribed for a person with Type 2 Diabetes. But many doctors, swayed by drug company hype, prescribe metformin in the form of combination pills like Janumet or Synjardy that cost 15 times what metformin alone costs and include relatively untested drugs that have serious side effects.

You will be much safer taking the plain generic metformin rather than one of these combos. In addition, the combo pills, because they include two different drugs whose dosage is fixed, may make it impossible to adjust the metformin dose to the size that is right for you without taking a large dose of the other drug.

What Metformin Does

Metformin Stops Liver Glucose Dumping

There is some scholarly debate about what exactly it is that metformin really does, but most researchers agree that, for most people, metformin limits the ability of the liver to convert glycogen into glucose and dump it into the bloodstream.

If you'll remember, an insulin resistant liver's tendency to keep dumping additional glucose into the bloodstream at mealtimes, when glucose from a meal is also coming in, can drive blood sugar way up after eating. The liver may also dump extra glucose in the bloodstream early in the morning when fasting insulin levels are low. So many people find that metformin lowers their fasting blood sugar as well as their post-meal blood sugars.

A mouse study published in 2009 suggests that metformin lowers blood sugar in the liver by directly stimulating a gene in the liver that shuts off glucose production.

Metformin Activates AMP Kinase

At the same time, metformin also activates an enzyme, AMP Kinase, which is present in muscle, liver, and heart cells. Because this enzyme is usually activated only after exercise has burnt off muscle energy stores, metformin, in effect, tricks your muscles and liver into behaving as if you had just exercised. They stop converting glucose into fat and switch into a fat burning mode. One last beneficial result of the way metformin stimulates AMP Kinase is that this enzyme also appears to protect the heart muscle during a heart attack.

Metformin May Boost GLP-1 Level

GLP-1 is a hormone secreted in the gut. It appears to stimulate insulin release when blood sugars rise. It also limits the production of the pancreatic hormone that is insulin's opposite, **glucagon**, a hormone that raises blood sugars. We will be discussing GLP-1 at length in the next chapter when we discuss the incretin drugs, which are designed to manipulate GLP-1 levels. But some little known research suggests that metformin also raises the level of GLP-1 after meals.

However, unlike the incretin drugs, metformin only raises GLP-1 levels in the post-meal period, avoiding the problems associated with incretin drugs that may keep it higher at all times.

Metformin Appears to Protect Against Heart Disease

This idea has been floating around for years, though it has only been in the last few years that researchers have gained insight into why it might be true. It turns out that one way metformin fights heart disease is by improving the function of the endothelium—the lining of the blood vessels. Patients who took metformin for roughly 4 years experienced highly significant drops in plasma levels of a long list of proteins associated with blood vessel inflammation. Since the other generic oral drugs commonly prescribed for diabetes have either been linked to increased heart attacks (sulfonylureas) or can lead to heart failure (Avandia and Actos) this data should reinforce the idea that metformin is the safest of the oral diabetic drugs and the one most likely to improve health outcomes over the long term.

Metformin May Also Fight Cancer

Intriguing data began emerging in 2009 suggesting that metformin has cancer fighting abilities that go beyond its ability to lower insulin resistance. Several studies have shown that people with diabetes who take metformin for a decade have less likelihood of developing cancers than people with diabetes who don't. One of these, a study published in 2010, found that the cancer risk of people with diabetes taking metformin was identical to that of the population at large, though those who didn't take it had a higher than normal risk. This was significant because before this study was published all earlier studies had suggested that people with diabetes have a *higher* risk of cancer than normal people. This was attributed to cancer cells' affinity for glucose.

However, another large epidemiological study published in 2014 found no difference in the incidence of cancer between patients in the UK who were taking metformin and those taking a sulfonylurea drug.

Even so, there is intriguing evidence that metformin might be helpful against specific kinds of cancer. A rodent study found that metformin stops breast cancer stem cells from growing. Another study, published in 2011 and conducted in women with PCOS, found that six months of treatment with metformin decreased the invasiveness of endometrial cancer cells by 25% compared to the activity of the same cells in women with PCOS who had not taken metformin.

What exactly metformin might be doing to combat breast cancer was shown by an analysis of data from the Women's Health Initiative study. It found that, though overall there was no difference in breast cancer incidence between the women with diabetes in the study and women without it, women with diabetes who were treated with metformin had a lower incidence of *invasive* breast cancer and fewer hormone sensitive cancers than did any of the women who weren't taking the drug, even those with normal blood sugars. The same study showed that women with diabetes who were treated with medications *other* than metformin had a slightly higher breast cancer incidence than women who did not have diabetes.

Metformin Lowers Risk of *All* Kinds of Fatal Outcomes

A study presented at the 2010 ADA Scientific Sessions analyzed records of "19,699 patients over age 45 who had diabetes as well as documented cardiovascular disease or other atherothrombotic [relating to blood clots in blood vessels] risk factors." It found that "... patients on metformin had a significant 33% reduction in the risk of death compared with those not on the drug." Even after the researchers adjusted their findings to account for other heart-protective drugs these patients were taking they still found a "24% reduction in death."

People on Metformin Live Slightly Longer than Normal People

An epidemiological study published in 2014 analyzed data from "78,241 subjects treated with metformin, 12,222 treated with sulfonylurea [glipizide, glyburide, etc], and 90,463 matched subjects without diabetes, whose data was in the UK Clinical Practice Research Datalink. They concluded that,

> Patients with type 2 diabetes initiated with metformin monotherapy had longer survival than did matched, non-diabetic controls. ... This supports the position of metformin as first-line therapy and implies that metformin may confer benefit in non-diabetes.

Adjusted for "relevant co-variables," the study reported that "adjusted median survival time" of people without diabetes in the study was 15% lower than that of people with diabetes taking metformin, while the adjusted mean survival time of people with diabetes taking sulfonylurea drugs was 38% lower.

Metformin's Effect on High Blood Sugar

This is all very well and good, but by now you may be wondering what, if anything, will metformin do for your blood sugar?

A follow-up study that tracked what happened to people participating in the UKPDS study after 20 years found that at the end of this period patients treated with metformin had a greater than 21% reduction in the risk of any "diabetes endpoint," i.e. complication, as well as a 30% reduction in risk of diabetes-related death.

That said, the incidence of complications and diabetes related deaths in the UKPDS study was still unacceptably high, because metformin alone cannot lower blood sugar to safe levels. The UKPDS researchers settled for A1cs in the 7% range, which as we saw earlier is high enough to guarantee heart disease and neuropathy.

In the manufacturer's Prescribing Information for metformin ER, a chart reports the results of a study that showed that for 141 diabetic subjects put on metformin, the average fasting plasma glucose dropped 53 mg/dl. However, the final fasting plasma glucose level in these subjects was still a whopping 189 mg/dl. No data is given in the Prescribing Information about the effect that metformin had on their post-challenge (i.e. post-OGTT) blood sugar concentrations.

A study performed by researchers at the University of Texas in 1991, which did examine post-challenge blood sugar, gave glucose tolerance tests to 14 diabetic patients taking metformin. The researchers found that metformin reduced the average OGTT two hour result from 360 mg/dl to 306 mg/dl. This left the subjects with blood sugars that were still dangerously high. metformin also reduced the subjects' fasting blood sugars from an average of 207 mg/dl to 158 mg/dl. Again this still left them with a toxic blood sugar level.

Another, larger, study, which compared metformin with Avandia put 100 newly diagnosed people with diabetes on metformin and found that their average *fasting blood sugar* dropped from 223 mg/dl to 173 mg/dl, which is still far above the level that might prevent complications. That study did not measure two hour OGTT values, but since the participants' A1cs dropped only to 7.1%, which correlates with an average blood sugar of 175 mg/dl, they were most certainly still dangerously elevated.

This makes it clear that you should not expect metformin alone to drop either your fasting blood sugar or your post-meal blood sugars more than roughly 50 mg/dl.

There's No Research Data About the Effect of Combining Metformin with Carbohydrate Restriction

Though the 50 mg/dl drop documented above doesn't sound like it would make much of an improvement to most people's diabetic blood sugars, anecdotal reports suggest that metformin does a much better job of lowering blood sugar in people who limit their carbohydrate intake than it does in people eating the high carbohydrate/low fat diets used in studies.

Metformin can also be helpful for people trying to lose weight. Messages posted on web discussion groups suggest that people who have a lot of weight to lose, whose weight loss has stalled out on a long-term low carbohydrate diet, often start losing again when they add metformin to their low carbohydrate diet regimen.

Others people report that when they take metformin while eating a low carbohydrate diet they can eat slightly more carbohydrate per meal without spiking. Others report that it lowers their fasting blood sugar but not their post-meal numbers. The explanation for these differences probably lies in the differing underlying causes of their diabetes. Some people find that metformin decreases their appetite, which also helps with weight loss. Metformin may also make it easier to keep from gaining weight, especially for insulin resistant people who use injected insulin.

Starting Metformin Early Is Far More Effective than Starting Later

A study published in 2010, of 1,799 Kaiser patients who were able to lower their A1c below 7.5% using metformin found that when patients were started on metformin immediately after diagnosis they were able to stay at an A1c lower than 7% for longer than did patients whose doctors waited a year before starting them on the drug.

This is important, since many people with diabetes resist taking a drug when they are first diagnosed, thinking that it is better to attempt to lower blood sugar with diet or exercise alone.

But because the overall effect of metformin differs from the effects of cutting carbs or exercising, this may be a mistake. It may be better to start metformin along with other approaches as soon as you receive a diagnosis of any form of abnormal blood sugar including prediabetes, rather than waiting.

What You Need To Know About Taking Metformin

Metformin comes in an extended release (ER) form taken once a day and a plain form taken three times a day at meals. Metformin in either form takes about three days to start working and two weeks to achieve its maximum effect. Because it often causes nausea and diarrhea during the first weeks as your body adjusts to it, it's advisable to start out with a low dose and work up. Most people don't see an effect on blood sugars until they are taking between 1,000 and 1,500 mg a day. Larger people may need to take the full dose (2250 to 2500 mg depending on whether they take metformin ER or plain metformin.)

Timing when you take metformin ER will often subtly change the impact it has on your blood sugar, because even the extended release form does not result in a completely smooth activity curve. Taking metformin ER at night will often result in a stronger effect on fasting blood sugar but less effect at dinner. Taking metformin ER in the morning may give best coverage on lunch, decent coverage for dinner, but result in the highest fasting blood sugars and the most stomach discomfort. You can experiment with the time you take metformin as long as you *never* take more than the prescribed dose during a 24 hour period.

Metformin Side Effects

Gastric Distress

The most common side effects of metformin are nausea, diarrhea, heartburn, and gas. That's why it's been nicknamed "metfartin" by people who post on web bulletin boards. These unpleasant digestive system symptoms often go away after a few weeks, but not always. Some people are unable to take metformin because of the persistence of these symptoms.

The plain form taken at meals is often harder to tolerate, so switching to the extended release form of metformin may relieve gastric symptoms.

Many of us also find that taking metformin ER in the early afternoon after we have eaten several meals may eliminate heartburn or the stomach irritation that occurs when it is taken on a relatively empty stomach.

If your problem is gas or diarrhea, try eating less starch. These symptoms may be caused by undigested starches reaching the gut where they are fermented by helpful bacteria.

However, another reason why you may experience gastric problems with metformin is that many pharmacies dispense whatever generic brand is cheapest in order to maximize their profits. My experience has been that several of these cheaper brands cause much more nausea and digestive distress than others. If you don't adapt to metformin within a month, ask the pharmacist to fill your prescription with a different generic brand. If they refuse, use another pharmacy. Even if your insurer forces you to use one pharmacy, metformin is so cheap that you can often find another pharmacy that will sell you a month's supply, without insurance, for no more than the copay you pay with insurance.

Does Metformin Cause Lactic Acidosis?

Metformin is chemically similar to an earlier drug, Phenformin, which was taken off the market because it caused a fatal side effect, lactic acidosis. So there was concern after metformin was approved that it, too, might cause lactic acidosis. However, subsequent research has established that lactic acidosis is very rare, and that people taking metformin don't experience it at rates higher than the general population. It also turns out that people with diabetes taking metformin have slightly *less* lactic acidosis than people taking sulfonylurea drugs.

When lactic acidosis does occur, it appears to be caused by what researchers call "concurrent comorbidity" which means another medical problem — usually kidney disease. This is why people with kidney damage, liver damage, or congestive heart failure should not take metformin.

Lactic Acidosis can also occur with dehydration in people who have otherwise normal kidney and liver function. If you develop a truly dehydrating condition like severe diarrhea, stop your metformin until you recover. You should also stop taking metformin a few days before and after you have X-rays with an injected contrast medium as the chemicals used in the contrast media may temporarily weaken kidney function.

Because abnormal kidney function and/or dehydration raise the risk of lactic acidosis, it may be a bad idea to take metformin with the new SGLT2 inhibitor diabetes drugs. We will be discussing these drugs in the next chapter.

Overindulging in alcohol may damage the liver in ways that also may enhance the risk of lactic acidosis, so people taking metformin are advised not to drink more than a very small amount of alcohol.

Metformin May Deplete Vitamin B-12 and Folate

Metformin has one more significant side effect. It may deplete Vitamin B-12 because it can alter the ability to absorb vitamin B-12 from the gut. If this is the case, oral supplementation will not help, as your body will not be able to absorb the vitamin as it passes through your body. You would need to have Vitamin B-12 shots to address this deficiency.

Typically it takes about 10 years for low Vitamin B-12 levels to develop, but if you are already marginal for Vitamin B-12 or have other issues with your ability to absorb nutrients this might happen earlier. Your doctor should periodically test your Vitamin B-12 levels if you are taking metformin.

Low vitamin B-12 can cause an irreversible form of neuropathy that can be confused with diabetic neuropathy. If you develop symptoms of neuropathy after years of taking metformin, don't assume it has been caused by your diabetes, even if your doctor suggests this is the case. Instead, insist on having your blood levels of B-12 measured.

Research Flags Metformin Both as a Cause and Cure for Dementia

There is conflicting evidence as to whether metformin raises the risk of dementia in people with diabetes or lowers it. Quite a few studies provide support for either argument. But a scholarly review of these studies, published in 2014, concluded that none of the studies conducted in humans went into enough detail to be able to rule out the potential influence of treatment protocol differences or the dozens of other genetic and lifestyle factors that might have affected their results.

In the case of one large epidemiological study linking metformin to dementia, conducted in Australia, some researchers suggest that the low vitamin B-12 levels associated with long-term metformin use may explain the findings of a higher rate of dementia in those taking metformin. This is another reason to get your B-12 levels checked every few years.

Acarbose: The Overlooked Diabetes Drug

Acarbose, a generic drug also sold under the brand name Precose, is a neglected but useful drug for controlling blood sugar. Like metformin, it has been the subject of a large study to see if it can prevent subjects from progressing from prediabetes to full-fledged diabetes. Though it has long been prescribed in Europe, it is rarely used in the United States and many doctors are unaware of how helpful it can be to people with either diabetes or impaired glucose tolerance.

How Acarbose Works

Acarbose works by blocking alpha-glucosidase, the enzyme that chops starches and complex sugars into their component glucose molecules. When this enzyme is blocked, starches and complex sugars pass through the stomach and portions of the small intestine largely undigested rather than entering the bloodstream as glucose.

However, acarbose is not that mythical substance so beloved by health scammers, the "starch blocker." Most of the starch and sugar whose digestion is temporarily blocked by acarbose does, eventually, get broken down into glucose by the bacteria that live in the gut. Then that glucose reaches the bloodstream. However, because the digestive process is slowed down, glucose reaches the bloodstream in dribs and drabs rather than in one big blood sugar-spiking dump.

How Much Improvement Does Acarbose Make in Blood Sugar?

The Prescribing Information provided by Bayer, the manufacturer of the Precose brand of acarbose, reports that in clinical trials Precose lowered post-meal blood sugar numbers by 25 mg/dl to 83 mg/dl depending on dosage. At the most commonly prescribed dose, Precose caused a drop of 46 mg/dl. The same Prescribing Information insert also reports that, in another study, subjects taking 100 mg of Precose at meals over four months experienced an average drop in one hour post-meal numbers of 42.6 mg/dl.

Unfortunately, none of these studies reported the amount of carbohydrate that patients ate when they achieved these improvements. In one study published by Bayer the baseline one hour post-meal blood sugar of the subjects was a hefty 299.1 mg/dl, so even with the Precose, these study subjects were running blood sugars that were dangerously high. Animal studies conducted throughout the 1990s suggested that even though this reduction in blood sugar was modest, acarbose also decreased protein glycation and appeared to delay or prevent heart attacks and the other diabetic complications caused by elevated blood sugars.

Does Acarbose Prevent the Development of Diabetes?

To see if acarbose could be used to prevent the progression of impaired glucose tolerance to diabetes, the multiple research centers that conducted the STOP-NIDDM Trial administered 100 mg of acarbose three times a day to 714 subjects while giving another 715 subjects a placebo. At the end of three years a smaller percentage of the group taking acarbose had developed diabetes than of the controls. The researchers concluded this meant acarbose could significantly decrease the progress of IGT to diabetes. In addition, the people taking acarbose appeared to have half as great a risk of cardiovascular events (heart attack, death, heart failure, stroke, or peripheral vascular disease) as controls. They also developed fewer new cases of hypertension.

However, these conclusions were called into question by a review of the study, which suggested that the results may have been manipulated by researchers connected to the drug's manufacturer.

Acarbose and a Carb-Restricted Diet

There are no studies that look at what happens when people who are already controlling their carbohydrate intake use acarbose to achieve healthy blood sugar targets. Anecdotal evidence suggests that when people eating a carb-restricted diet use acarbose to allow them to add an occasional high carbohydrate indulgence to their diet, it can be helpful.

However, acarbose does not allow you to totally pig out. Eating more than an extra 20-30 grams of carbohydrate per meal with acarbose may cause you to experience high blood sugar spikes three or four hours after eating, since that is when the starches and sugars will finally digest. The height of those spikes will depend on how much second-phase insulin release you have left.

Acarbose Does Not Block Simple Sugars

If you are using acarbose, it is important to understand that it does not slow the digestion of simple sugars, because they do not require digestion but are absorbed from the stomach as soon as they are eaten.

Thus sweeteners containing pure glucose like honey, maple syrup, or candies made with dextrose will go straight into your bloodstream, whether you have taken acarbose or not. Acarbose works well with sucrose — table sugar — and starches like wheat flour, rice, and beans.

Dosing and Time to Take Effect

You should start out taking the lowest dose of acarbose available and then work up. This will help you avoid gastric side effects. You take acarbose with your first bite of food and it begins to work immediately. Unlike other drugs, acarbose does not get into your body in any significant amounts. It exerts its effect within the digestive tract and is not absorbed.

Gas—the Killer Side Effect of Acarbose

Fully 24% of the people assigned to the acarbose group in the STOP-NIDDM study dropped out of the study long before it completed. There's a reason for this. When undigested carbohydrate travels through your digestive tract the so-called friendly bacteria digest it. That kind of "digestion" also goes by the name of "fermentation" and one of its byproducts is gas.

This means that the more carbohydrates you eat with acarbose, the more gas will be produced in your gut. The resulting gas production can be intense enough to limit your social life—or motivate you to cut down on your carbohydrate intake very steeply, since you quickly learn to associate high carbohydrate dinners with hours of post-meal flatulence. However, if you eat a more modest carbohydrate intake with acarbose, it can be useful.

Combining Acarbose and Metformin

Adding acarbose to metformin helps you achieve even better blood sugar control. However, I have also found it is better to use a lower dose of metformin (500 mg/day) along with a lower dose of acarbose (50 mg), since combining these drugs really ramps up the gas and gastric misery. Taking both drugs at a high dose simultaneously can result in acute stomach distress.

Drugs that Stimulate Insulin Secretion

The drugs we've discussed up until now lower blood sugar by keeping glucose from going into the blood stream or encouraging the muscles to remove it from the blood. There is another group of oral antidiabetic drugs, which lower blood sugar by forcing the beta cells to produce more insulin.

There are two families of these drugs: the **sulfonylurea drugs**, which include glipizide (brand names Glucotrol and Glucotrol XL), glyburide/glibenclamide (Micronase, Glynase, and DiaBeta), gliclazide (Diamicron, not sold in the United States) and glimepiride (Amaryl) and the newer family of **meglitinide** or "glinide" drugs, which include nateglinide (brand name, Starlix) and repaglinide

(Prandin).

The sulfonylurea drugs were the very first oral diabetes drugs. They were first sold in the United States in the 1970s and were the only oral diabetic drugs available in the United States until the mid-1990s. Today they are among the cheapest generic drugs available for Type 2 diabetes and are still widely prescribed, especially by family doctors.

The glinide drugs have only become available in cheaper generic versions within the past few years. Far fewer doctors prescribe them instead of the older sulfonylureas, though they are safer and less likely to cause hypos.

Sulfonylurea Drugs Stimulate Insulin Production for 8-12 hours Regardless of Blood Sugar Level

The sulfonylurea drugs bind to an ATP-dependent K+ (KATP) channel in the beta cell membrane, which causes the beta cell to steadily secrete insulin whether or not glucose is present in the blood stream. The effect lasts from eight to twelve hours. Because of this, these drugs are notorious for causing dangerous hypos.

That's why people who take these drugs are often advised to keep their carbohydrate consumption high to avoid dangerous hypoglycemic episodes. Since our goal is to lower blood sugar, that rules these drugs out as useful tools since they require that patients maintain their blood sugar at levels far above 140 mg/dl in order to avoid hypos.

The Short-Acting Meglitinides, Repaglinide and Nateglinide

These two drugs also work on the ATP-dependent K+ (KATP) channel of the beta cell membrane, but at a different site. They have a half life within the body of only 1-1.5 hours, and they are usually done lowering blood sugar by three hours after they are taken. So if taken with meals, these drugs are less likely to cause hypos. Nevertheless, users of the glinide drugs report that they are still capable of causing hypos when too high a dose is taken or when taken with meals low in carbohydrate.

The Meglitinide Drugs May Also Raise GLP-1 by Inhibiting DPP-4

A study shows that repaglinide and Nateglinide appear to inhibit an enzyme, DPP-4, in a manner similar to Januvia. We will discuss DPP-4 inhibition in the next chapter when we discuss the incretin drugs. For now, note that because these drugs have a much shorter half-life in the body—1.5 and 1 hours vs. 12.5 hours for Januvia—their suppression of DPP-4 may be short-term, which would make them less likely to cause the dangerous side effects of incretin drugs.

Most Sulfonylurea Drugs Raise Heart Attack Risk

Sulfonylurea drugs have been found to raise the incidence of heart attack. This is because they not only stimulate the beta cells, they also stimulate a receptor on the heart muscle.

Drug companies insisted that this was only true of the older, first generation sulfonylurea drugs, but a study analyzing the health records of all Danish residents over 20 years old who took either a sulfonylurea, a glinide, or metformin between 1997 and 2006 found that only repaglinide and the sulfonylurea drug gliclazide, which is not sold in the United States, were as safe as metformin.

All the other sulfonylurea drugs raised the risk of death, whether or not people had had a heart attack before taking them. The study concluded:

> Monotherapy with the most used I[nsulin]S[ecretagogues]s, including glimepiride, glibenclamide, glipizide, and tolbutamide, seems to be associated with increased mortality and cardiovascular risk compared with metformin. Gliclazide and repaglinide appear to be associated with a lower risk than other I[nsulin]S[ecretagogues]s.

The UKPDS 10 year follow-up study also shows that sulfonylurea drugs are a poor choice compared to metformin. It found that patients in the Sulfonylurea-insulin group had only a 9% risk reduction in any diabetes-related endpoint compared to the 21% risk reduction experienced by those taking metformin. Their risk of death due to diabetes was reduced by only 17% compared to the 30% risk reduction seen in those taking metformin.

Since gliclazide, the one safe sulfonylurea drug, is not sold in the United States, the only safe choice for Americans who need a drug that stimulates insulin production is repaglinide.

Combining Insulin Stimulating Drugs with Others Causes Hypos

The FDA has issued updates to the prescribing information for glimepiride and other sulfonylureas as well as for repaglinide, warning that their blood sugar lowering effect may be magnified when they are taken with other medications that slow their removal from the body. This may allow them cause dangerous hypos.

The drugs that were already known to interact with sulfonylureas are: nonsteroidal anti-inflammatory drugs (Motrin, Advil, and Ibuprofen), clarithromycin, and other drugs that are highly protein bound, such as salicylates (aspirin and salsalate), sulfonamides antibiotics (Bactrim/Septra), chloramphenicol, coumarins, probenecid, monoamine oxidase inhibitors, and ß-adrenergic blocking agents.

To this list the FDA has added disopyramide (Norpace), fluoxetine

(Prozac), and the quinolone antibiotics (Cipro, Noroxin, Levaquin etc.), all of which also potentiate the effects of sulfonylureas.

The warnings for repaglinide now include gemfibrozil (Lopid) and the immune suppressor cyclosporin.

Because doctors aren't always aware of these drug interactions, if you are prescribed any of these insulin stimulating drugs, check with your pharmacist to make sure that you aren't taking another drug that could make you more likely to suffer dangerous hypos.

Combining Repaglinide with Metformin Can Amplify its Impact

Combining repaglinide with metformin can greatly amplify the impact of *both* drugs on blood sugar. The Prandin Prescribing Information reveals that over a 4-5 month period, people taking repaglinide alone saw their fasting blood sugar *rise* by an average of 8 mg/dl while people taking metformin alone saw an average *drop* in their fasting blood sugar of 4.5 mg/dl. But people taking *both* drugs simultaneously experienced an average decline in fasting blood sugar of *39.2 mg/dl* — almost ten times as much as with metformin alone!

In addition, some people taking repaglinide (including myself) have found that over time it can wear away the body's ability to raise blood sugars when they drop too low, resulting in the sudden onset of frighteningly low hypos. After 6 months of taking repaglinide and metformin without incident I experienced two hypos in the 40 mg/dl range within one week, though I had not changed my diet or dose. I have heard similar stories from others. If you see your fasting blood sugar dropping below the 80s while taking repaglinide, it may be time to lower your dose or to take a "drug vacation" for a few weeks to avoid experiencing dangerous hypos without warning.

Do Insulin Stimulating Drugs Cause Beta Cell Burnout?

There is some question about the wisdom of forcing already dysfunctional beta cells to produce yet more insulin. Dr. Richard K. Bernstein is a firm believer that these kinds of drugs cause beta cells to die and counsels people with diabetes to avoid them. However, there is little experimental data available to evaluate this possibility.

Some argue that UKPDS proved sulfonylurea drugs do not burn out beta cells since, in that study, those taking metformin and sulfonylurea drugs experienced the same gradual decrease in blood sugar control over the years.

A rodent study published in 2008 found that though long-term use of Glibenclamide caused mouse beta cells to stop secreting insulin, this effect was completely reversed as soon as the mice were taken off the drug, suggesting that their beta cells had remained intact while the drug was taken. This suggests that it is probably a good idea to take a drug vacation from these drugs if you see them losing their efficacy.

Of course, beta cells *will* be destroyed if the insulin-stimulating drug does not lower your blood sugars to a level low enough to prevent glucose toxicity, as often happens. So it is possible that the high blood sugars that are still experienced by people taking sulfonylurea drugs are what kill their beta cells rather than the drugs.

Insulin Stimulating Drugs Are Associated with Weight Gain

Drugs that stimulate insulin production are also known to cause weight gain. This may be because the insulin they secrete causes blood sugar to drop steeply, which, as we know, makes people hungry.

Thiazolidinediones: Rosiglitazone and Pioglitazone

Rosiglitazone (Brand name, Avandia) and pioglitazone (Actos) are two very similar drugs. They are members of the thiazolidinediones (TZD), family that was the hot new thing in diabetes treatment the early 2000s. They are now generic, as their patents have expired. Because almost two decades have passed since they came to market, doctors now have a much better idea of what they do than they did during the years when they were earning billions of dollars for their makers.

Three drugs in this class began their careers by showing great promise in the treatment of insulin resistance. When they first hit the market the drug companies touted preliminary research they claimed showed that these drugs might be able to regrow failing beta cells.

Unfortunately, over time all three TZDs were found to cause life-threatening side effects, the risk of which was far greater than the benefit these drugs provided. The hope that they might rescue failing beta cells also proved to be a mirage.

Rezulin, the first of these drugs and the one that endocrinologists tell me was by far the most effective, was withdrawn after it was found to cause fatal liver failure in a small but significant number of patients. Avandia and Actos came to market in the late 1990s with the promise that they did not cause liver failure—though post-marketing reports later discovered that this was not entirely true as there are reports of liver failure associated with these drugs.

But it took more than a decade for the real problems with these drugs to surface. It was not until shortly before the patent for Avandia expired in 2012 that the public was made aware of the many significant problems with these drugs that researchers had known about for many years. However, readers of my blog and web site would have already learned about some of these problems, since I had read about them in obscure publications that flagged them.

Once the patents expired, the big money had been made and the salespeople moved on. So you are less likely to be prescribed one of these drugs now that they are available in the form of cheap generics. But some family doctors who have prescribed them for years are still prescribing them.

What These Drugs Do

These drugs supposedly decrease insulin resistance. This sounds exciting until you learn that they do this by causing the formation of new fat cells, primarily on the arms, thighs, and butt, into which insulin pushes excess glucose taken from the bloodstream.

Like the other, safer, oral diabetes drugs discussed earlier in this chapter, the manufacturer's own official Prescribing Information makes it clear that whatever it is that they do, the TZDs produce only a modest change in blood sugar and insulin levels, though some research suggests they may produce slightly better blood sugars than metformin does.

Beta Cell Rest Proved to Be a Myth

Because research showed that Actos preserved the beta cell islet structure in two strains of diabetic mice whose diabetes was caused by damaging a specific gene, the drug's manufacturer raised hopes that it might do something similar for people. The premise that both Actos and Avandia could rejuvenate beta cells was promoted so effectively by drug company salespeople that many doctors told patients to keep taking these drugs to revive beta cells, even when they experienced serious side effects and saw little effect on their blood sugars.

But the hope that TZD drugs could rejuvenate beta cells was dashed by the publication in 2007 of the results from a large study of Avandia. The study, called DREAM, went on to become a nightmare for those taking the drug. DREAM had initially appeared to show that taking Avandia could prevent the onset of diabetes—but a follow-up study found that as soon as the drug was stopped, people developed diabetes at the same rate as if they hadn't taken the drug. This made it crystal clear that the claim that these drugs helped beta cells heal themselves was not true. Had beta cells been rejuvenated, blood sugar response would have been improved after the drug was discontinued.

Avandia Appears to Promote Heart Attack

That was just the beginning of the bad news that came out of the DREAM study. The study had been funded by Avandia's manufacturer, GlaxoSmithWellcome, in the hope that it would prove that Avandia would prevent heart disease. Instead it found the opposite.

Patients who took Avandia had 66% percent more heart attacks, 39% more strokes, and 20% more deaths from cardiovascular related problems than those who did not.

Then the news came out that in 1999 Glaxo had silenced an early critic of Avandia who had uncovered evidence pointing to Avandia's connection with heart problems. The drug company had shut him up by threatening to bring an expensive law suit against the critic's university. The threat was effective and the scientist did not make public the information he had about Avandia's possible role in causing heart attacks. Only in 2007 did FDA drug reviewers finally publish a report confirming that patients taking Avandia are more likely to suffer and die from heart problems than those taking Actos.

In 2013 the maker of Avandia managed to convince the FDA that reanalysis of yet another study proved that Avandia did not cause excess heart attacks. and the FDA removed restraints on prescribing it. However, Dr. Steven Nissen, a very high profile cardiologist from the Cleveland Clinic, who was one of the investigators behind the studies that originally pointed to an elevated risk with Avandia, told the Associated Press, that this was an attempt by the FDA to save face, explaining, "This is about appearances, not changing medical practice. A single reanalysis of a trial does not exonerate a drug where all the other data point to increased cardiovascular risks."

Actos is Not Very Effective and Causes Heart Failure

When the bad news about Avandia finally reached the public, doctors switched many of their patients to Actos. However, a meta-study published in 2006 which analyzed the results of 22 randomized clinical trials involving 6,200 patients with Type 2 Diabetes who took Actos concluded that,

> ... published scientific studies of at least 24 weeks of pioglitazone [Actos] treatment in people with Type 2 Diabetes mellitus did not provide convincing evidence that patient-oriented outcomes like mortality, morbidity, adverse effects and health-related quality of life are positively influenced by this drug. Until new evidence becomes available, the benefit-risk ratio of pioglitazone [Actos] therapy in Type 2 Diabetes mellitus remains unclear.

According to Dr Richter, the author of this study, not only did the review find no clear-cut benefit to using Actos, but it also showed an increased occurrence of edema [water swelling] and heart failure — including heart failure requiring hospital admission — among patients taking the drug.

Actos's patent expires in 2016. When it does, you will probably see a spate of new research published documenting the problems with this drug. But until it is off patent, research institutions are not likely to alienate the company still earning a good income from it.

Actos and Avandia Grow New and Permanent Fat Cells

Aside from their ability to cause dangerous water retention, Actos and Avandia make people fatter. It has long been known that all the drugs in the thiazolidinedione family cause weight gain. Because they also cause the water retention and swelling that now are linked with heart failure, it was first believed that this weight gain attributed to these drugs was caused solely by water retention.

When it was later determined that *real fat* was being deposited on the bodies of those taking it, the drug companies spun this information by claiming that in people taking the drug the hip/waist ratio had changed. They suggested this might be because abdominal fat—the kind known to correlate with insulin resistance—was decreasing, which would be a good thing.

However, when a group of researchers randomized a group of nondiabetic insulin resistant volunteers to either diet and exercise or Actos, they discovered that the *decrease in waist hip ratio that study subjects experienced while taking Actos was due to the increase in the size of their hips, not a decrease in their waists.*

The study found that Actos was causing an increase in the number of fat cells accumulating in what was euphemistically called "the lower body depot," an area most of us would probably recognize better when called by its common name: the butt. This is troubling, because once you add new fat cells they do not go away even when you diet. And the link between these drugs and a significant gain in body fat may have another cause, too. A rodent study published in 2015 found evidence that these drugs may also cause weight gain by increasing hunger levels in the brain.

Calorie Restriction and Exercise Work Better than TZDs

It is even more troubling to learn that the blood sugar improvements Actos made in the study subjects taking it could have been achieved without adding new fat cells to their butts. The group of insulin resistant volunteers in the study just cited who took *no drug* but cut 500 calories a day from their diet and exercised for 45 minutes a day achieved far better improvements in their fasting insulin levels, their fasting triglyceride levels, and their total cholesterol than did the Actos group—while losing weight from both their waists and their "lower body depot."

Other Serious Side Effects of Actos and Avandia

Heart Failure When Taken with Any Insulin

The Prescribing Information for all the insulins currently on the market warn that taking TZDs (Actos or Avandia) with insulin can cause fluid retention and heart failure.

Macular Edema

Another dangerous side effect that has been associated with both TZD drugs is macular edema—swelling in the retina, which can lead to blindness. This swelling does not always resolve when the drug is discontinued. A study published in 2009 which analyzed the records of 170,000 people with diabetes treated by Kaiser Permanente Southern California, found that people taking TZD drugs—most of whom were taking Actos—were 60% more likely to develop Macular Edema, even with well-controlled blood sugars, than people not taking a TDZ drug.

Liver Toxicity

Despite the original claim that they were not toxic to the liver, there have been a few reports of liver disease occurring in patients taking these drugs. While it does appear they are less damaging than Rezulin, they do raise liver enzymes, which often means that liver damage is occurring. Experts suggest that monitoring liver enzymes may not be enough to prevent damage.

Fractures with Both Avandia and Actos

Several studies have shown that people of both genders and all ages are more likely to experience broken bones after taking Actos or Avandia for several years. One study published in the *New England Journal of Medicine* compared Avandia to metformin and glyburide and found twice as many bone fractures in the group of patients taking Avandia. A meta-analysis published in 2008 concluded that use of Avandia or Actos doubled a woman's risk of fracture.

In discussing this study one of the researchers was reported as saying,

> .. if thiazolidinediones (TZDs) are used by elderly, postmenopausal women (around 70 years) with type 2 diabetes for one year, one additional fracture would occur among every 21 women. Among younger women (around 56 years), use of the drugs for one year or longer would result in one additional fracture for every 55 women.

This finding was confirmed by another study that analyzed the medical records of 19,070 patients. It found a 57% higher risk of fractures in women of all ages and a 71% higher risk in post-menopausal women taking Actos or Avandia.

The mechanism by which these drugs cause fractures appears to be that they create new fat cells by causing the cells that are supposed to turn into new bone cells to turn into new fat cells instead. Deprived of the new bone they need for repair, bones become porous.

The reason that broken bones are more common among older women in these studies may be that they already have less bone mass than younger women or men, so any additional deterioration in their bones is more obvious. Over decades of use, bone brittleness may become a problem for *anyone* taking a TZD drug, no matter what their gender or age when starting it.

Actos Is Associated with a Higher Rate of Bladder Cancer

On Sept 17, 2010, the FDA announced that it was conducting a safety review of Actos, because preliminary (5 year) results from a 10 year study found

> ... there was an increased risk of bladder cancer in patients with the longest exposure to Actos and in those with the highest cumulative dose of the drug.

In June of 2011 the FDA confirmed that there was a heightened risk of bladder cancer with Actos.

Chapter Nine
Patented Diabetes Drugs

The drugs we discussed in the previous chapter have been prescribed for decades and their properties are well understood. Now it's time to examine the newer drugs that doctors are likely to prescribe when you can't lower your blood sugar with diet and exercise alone. Unlike the older drugs, these drugs are protected by patents and actively marketed by their manufacturers. They are the drugs you see advertised in magazines and on TV.

Because these new, patented drugs can earn billions of dollars, drug companies promote them with huge advertising budgets. Some of this money buys the ads you see in the media. A lot more pays for the drug company salespeople who visit doctors all around the country, bringing them free restaurant lunches and, of course, the latest sales pitches. A big slice of the ad budget covers the huge consulting and speaking fees paid to a coterie of high profile doctors who sing the praises of these new drugs in medical journals and newsletters. They also deliver lectures about them to their peers at professional get-togethers ranging in size from cozy local dinners to crowded national and international medical conferences.

Though people with diabetes living in countries outside of the United States don't have to worry about their doctors being influenced by salespeople bearing free lunches, the testimony of high profile company-paid doctors influences prescribing behavior around the world, even in countries with state-funded health care. And when problems do emerge with these drugs, the "expert" doctors on the corporate payrolls are the first to defend them and downplay any concerns raised by researchers—often without revealing to the media that they are on drug company payrolls.

There are several families of these new diabetes drugs, and within each family there are several competing medications, each sold by a different drug company. In this chapter, we will examine exactly what it is that these new drugs do. We will also take a hard look at the many serious problems that are already known to be associated with them.

Keep in mind, though, that, as we saw in the previous chapter, many of the most serious problems with profitable, patented drugs emerge only after they have been on sale for a decade or more—right before their patents—and profits—are due to expire. So if you decide to take any new drug, check online every few months to see if the FDA has issued any advisory bulletins about it. Our blog tracking changes to the Blood Sugar 101 web site also flags major issues that have arisen with all diabetes drugs. You'll find it at:

http://phlauntdiabetesupdates.blogspot.com/.

To help you keep track of which drug is which, we have provided a table listing these drugs by family and brand name in Appendix C.

The Incretin Drugs

The patented new diabetes drugs you are most likely to be prescribed are those in the family of medications called **incretin drugs**. The first of these drugs was approved in the middle 2000s, though new drugs in this family have been approved as recently as 2015, and more are awaiting approval. There are two subfamilies of these drugs, the DPP-4 inhibitors, the most prescribed of which is Januvia, and the GLP-1 receptor agonists, of which the current bestseller is Victoza.

What All Incretin Drugs Do

Both subfamilies of incretin drugs amplify the effect of a hormone, **GLP-1** which is produced primarily in the human gut but also in a region of the brain. GLP-1 does many things, but the thing it does that makes it a useful target in treating diabetes is that it stimulates insulin secretion when food reaches the gut. Unlike the older insulin stimulating drugs, which we discussed in the previous chapter, GLP-1 only stimulates beta cells to secrete insulin when the concentration of glucose in the bloodstream rises above a certain threshold. This means that unlike the older insulin stimulating drugs incretin drugs do not cause hypos.

GLP-1 also lowers the production of glucagon at meal times. Glucagon is the hormone that makes the liver dump glucose into the bloodstream during fasting periods to keep blood sugar from dropping too low. But in many people with Type 2 Diabetes, especially those whose livers are insulin resistant, glucagon continues to stimulate the liver to dump glucose even during meals when blood sugar is already high and rising. So turning off glucagon secretion at mealtimes further lowers post-meal blood sugars.

Besides lowering blood sugar, GLP-1 also appears to regulate the stomach valves. When GLP-1 levels are high, the lower stomach valve does not open and a person will have a feeling of fullness after eating a small amount of food. This makes it easier to eat less and lose weight. Apart from its effect in the stomach, GLP-1 levels in the brain directly influence how the brain experiences hunger. High levels of GLP-1 can induce a kind of anorexia that makes food look unappealing.

The GLP-1 your body secretes naturally has a half life of only two minutes, as almost immediately after it is secreted an enzyme called DPP-4 starts breaking it down. What incretin drugs do is intervene in a way that keeps GLP-1 working for hours, not minutes. This can result in prolonged insulin secretion in people with diabetes whose beta cells are still capable of responding to stimulation. It also decreases hunger, which may lead to weight loss.

There are two subfamilies of incretin drugs. The most popular includes the drugs called **DPP-4 Inhibitors**. These come in the form of pills. The other subfamily of incretin drugs is made up of the drugs called **GLP-1 Receptor Agonists.** Currently these must all be injected, though efforts are underway to provide at least one in pill form.

DPP-4 Inhibitors Turn off an Enzyme that Destroys GLP-1

DPP-4 inhibitors work by turning off the gene that produces the enzyme that otherwise destroys GLP-1 a few minutes after it has been secreted. The enzyme (and sometimes the gene) is called DPP-4. When the gene is inhibited, little of the DPP-4 enzyme is made, and the concentration of GLP-1 in the body rises to a level that is three times as high as normal. It remains at that level for hours at a time. DPP-4 inhibitors also raise the level of a second, less important incretin hormone, GIP, which also stimulates insulin secretion and appears to play a role in regulating bone remodeling.

The most commonly prescribed DPP-4 inhibitors are Januvia (generic name, sitagliptin) and Onglyza (saxagliptin). Some other DPP-4 inhibitors are the drug whose generic name is linagliptin, which is marketed under the brand names Trajenta, Tradjenta, Trayenta, and Trazenta in different parts of the world, and Nesina (generic name, alogliptin). As you have probably deduced by now, if a drug ends in "gliptin" it is likely to be a DPP-4 inhibitor.

Most DPP-4 inhibitors are also sold in a form that combines the expensive patented drug with metformin in one pill. These combo drugs include Janumet (Januvia and metformin), Kombiglyze (Onglyza and metformin), and Jentadueto (Trajenta and metformin).

GLP-1 Agonists Are Lab-Created Molecules that Mimic GLP-1

The other family of incretin drugs is made up of the **GLP-1 receptor agonists**. The word "agonist" is used when an artificially created molecule acts on a cell receptor the same way that a naturally occurring substance does. The GLP-1 agonists are lab-created proteins that are similar enough to natural GLP-1 that they activate the same cell receptors that natural GLP-1 does. However these artificially synthesized peptides are not chemically identical to GLP-1. They have been modified so that they resist being broken down. Therefore, unlike naturally produced GLP-1, they remain active in your body for hours or days, not minutes.

The bestselling GLP-1 receptor agonist has the generic name liraglutide. It is marketed under the name Victoza, when sold as a treatment for high blood sugar, and under the name Saxenda, when it is sold as a weight loss drug for people with normal blood sugar. Other members of the GLP-1 receptor agonist drug family include Byetta and its extended release form, Bydureon (generic name, exenatide), Trulicity (dulaglutide), Lyxumia (lixisenatide), and Tanzeum (albiglutide).

The first of the GLP-1 receptor agonists, Byetta, hit the market in 2005. Though it was touted as lowering blood sugar by stimulating insulin production, some anecdotal reports suggest that it actually lowered blood sugar primarily through its effect of keeping the valve at the bottom of the stomach shut, which slowed digestion long enough to allow second-phase insulin release to kick in and lower glucose. Several people who posted about their experiences with Byetta on the alt.support.diabetes newsgroup years ago reported that when taking Byetta they saw the blood sugar peaks they used to see at one and two hours after eating occurring three and four hours later.

The increasing use of these drugs for weight loss in people with normal blood sugars also suggests that their effect on insulin stimulation is minor. When Victoza was rebranded as a weight loss drug, not only was it renamed Saxenda, but its dosage was raised, even though it was being prescribed for people with normal blood sugars, who would be expected to experience dangerous low blood sugars if the higher dose of the drug stimulated more insulin secretion than the lower dose diabetes formulation does.

GLP-1 Agonists Work Well for a Subset of People with Diabetes

Studies of Byetta, the most effective of these drugs, found that one in four people who took it experienced significant weight loss, about 28 lbs each according to a press release from the drug's maker. Three in ten of those who took it saw their A1cs drop below 6.5%. However, more than half of those who took Byetta ended up with A1cs higher than 7% even after taking the drug for three years. This is still high enough to damage their organs. And the average weight loss for all those who took the drug over a three year period was only 11 pounds, in a population whose average starting weight was well over 200 lbs.

If you wonder why patients continued to inject themselves with an expensive drug, twice a day for three years, even though it produced such modest decreases in blood sugar and weight, the answer is this: just as happened with Avandia a decade earlier, drug company salespeople informed doctors that research had shown that Byetta could regrow failing beta cells. So patients continued using this seemingly ineffective drug because they were told it would heal their broken pancreases.

Similar claims were soon being made for Januvia, the first DPP-4 inhibitor to hit the market, which became the top bestselling non-psychiatric drug in the United States shortly after it was released. Even though a study cited in Januvia's own Prescribing Information showed that on average it only lowered the A1c of people who took it by a measly .6% —and that was in a group who started with an average A1c of 8% —doctors started prescribing Januvia to almost everyone with Type 2 Diabetes whose insurance would cover it, swayed by drug company salespeople who told them that research showed that incretin drugs increased the beta cell mass of animals that took them.

Although the official prescribing guidelines published by various professional organizations still state that the incretin drugs should not be prescribed until older, cheaper, and safer drugs have been tried, this aggressive marketing has ensured that most people Type 2 Diabetes are given an oral incretin drug shortly after diagnosis, as long as they have an insurance plan that will pay for its hefty cost. Many more, especially those desperate to lose weight, are prescribed injected GLP-1 receptor agonists. So these drugs continue to be among the most profitable ever sold. The bestselling DPP-4 inhibitor Januvia earned $3.9 billion in 2014. The bestselling GLP-1 Receptor agonist, Victoza, earned $2.3 billion —and this was before it was released under the name Saxenda as a weight loss drug.

However, studies have cast a sobering light on the claim that these drugs regrow functional beta cells. If that was true, you would expect that as time passed people taking these drugs would see improving blood sugar levels, as their shiny new beta cells made more and more insulin. But, in fact, the opposite has been observed. A follow-up study involving people originally enrolled in the Byetta drug acceptance trials found that their blood sugars, after initially improving, reached a plateau and then started to deteriorate again. Even at that plateau level, these patients still had fully diabetic blood sugars. And though Januvia has been in widespread use since 2006, no follow-up studies have demonstrated that the blood sugars of those taking it improve with longer use, either.

Incretin Drugs May Be Growing Highly Abnormal Pancreatic Cells

Meanwhile, worrisome data has emerged from quite a few unrelated animal and human studies performed by academic researchers not on drug company payrolls. It suggests that, while it is true that incretin drugs appear to be growing a lot of new cells in the pancreas, they are not growing the healthy, functional beta cells the salespeople have promised. Instead, incretin drugs appear to be growing abnormal pancreatic cells—both beta cells and glucagon-secreting alpha cells—that are forming abnormal and possibly invasive structures within the pancreas. These may, over time, cause severe and even potentially fatal side effects.

To protect their profits, the companies that sell these money makers have orchestrated very effective campaigns intended to cast doubt on the work of the highly respected researchers who have uncovered these problems. Their efforts are similar to what we saw happen with Avandia a decade earlier. The ADA, which is heavily funded by drug company money, has also actively taken steps to downplay the importance of this research, as it did with the research that linked Avandia to heart attack. As a result, most family doctors are not aware of these troubling findings and their implications for people taking incretin drugs. But the dangers are very real, and if you will be taking one of these drugs you need to know about them. Here is what we have learned so far about the abnormal cell growth that appears to occur in people who are taking incretin drugs.

Research Links Incretin Drugs to Changes in Pancreatic Cells

In 2009, the FDA issued a safety alert reporting that it had received reports linking Januvia to pancreatitis, a painful inflammation of the pancreas that can destroy large portions of it and lead to full-fledged Type 1 diabetes or even death. The drug's official prescribing information was amended to state, "There have been postmarketing reports of acute pancreatitis, including fatal and non-fatal hemorrhagic or necrotizing pancreatitis."

At the same time lab research was published that also suggested that DPP-4 inhibition might be causing abnormal cell growth in the pancreas. Reporting on their work with rats that had had human genes inserted into their pancreases, the researchers stated, "... sitagliptin [Januvia] treatment was associated with increased pancreatic ductal turnover, ductal metaplasia, and, in one rat, pancreatitis [emphasis mine]."

"Metaplasia" is defined in Mosby's Medical Dictionary as

> The reversible conversion of normal tissue cells into another, less differentiated cell type in response to chronic stress or injury. With prolonged exposure to the inducing stimulus, cancerous transformation can occur.

Aftermarket reports also linked Byetta, the first GLP-1 receptor agonist, to pancreatitis, too. To defuse these concerns, in 2010, Medco, a pharmacy benefits management company (now merged into Express

Scripts) published an analysis of its medical records, which claimed to find no increase in cases of pancreatitis among patients taking either Byetta or Januvia. This commercially-funded study appeared to prove that the rate of pancreatitis among people taking these drugs was identical to that of people with diabetes not taking them, though it was pointed out that the rate of pancreatitis was much higher in all the diabetic groups than in people without diabetes.

This finding was widely publicized, probably with the help of the salespeople for the companies selling these drugs. However, these studies were done at a time when the drugs were quite new and few patients had taken them for more than a few years. Given that small clusters of abnormal cells in the pancreas produce no symptoms and cannot be currently detected with any technique except the surgical removal of the pancreas, this result did not rule out the possibility that these drugs were causing dangerous changes in pancreatic cells.

Then, three years later in 2013, a second, more thorough, epidemiological study conducted by academic researchers at Johns Hopkins analyzed the medical records of over a million people with diabetes and reported:

> Our findings suggest a significantly increased risk of hospitalization for acute pancreatitis associated with the use of sitagliptin [Januvia] or exenatide [Byetta] among adult patients with type 2 diabetes mellitus. Our results support findings from mechanistic studies and spontaneous reports submitted to the US Food and Drug Association that such an association may be causal.

This study cast grave doubt on the claim based on the Medco research that pancreatitis was striking people with diabetes because they had diabetes, rather than because they were taking a specific drug.

Soon after the Johns Hopkins study was published, Dr. Peter Butler, a researcher at UCLA's David Geffen School of Medicine, published a research report that made clear why these drugs were causing an elevated risk of hospitalization for pancreatitis. Dr. Butler is one of very few experts in the difficult art of dissecting a human pancreas on autopsy—a process that is difficult because the digestive enzymes secreted by the organ tend to digest it at death. His report discussed autopsies he had done on the pancreases of 20 people with diabetes who had died of strokes and head injuries, which had left their pancreases undamaged. About half of these people had been taking an incretin drug for at least a year. All but one had been on Januvia, the other was on Byetta.

And yes, Dr. Butler found that these drugs do indeed appear to grow huge numbers of new beta cells and alpha cells in these people's pancreases. People with diabetes taking the incretin drugs had more than three times as much beta cell mass and alpha cell mass as people with diabetes not treated with incretin drugs. But the study also found that these cells were not growing in their normal patterns. They were found in "eccentrically shaped islets" and "in association with duct structures." The overgrowth of alpha and beta cells was described as "... encircling and sometimes encroaching on pancreatic ducts." These cells were growing into the ducts in ways that matched the changes seen in pancreatitis.

The people taking these incretin drugs were also found to have tiny glandular tumors scattered throughout their pancreases. Most of the tumors found in people taking Januvia were adenomas—a type of glandular tumor that starts out benign but can over time turn cancerous. A one centimeter neuroendocrine tumor was also found in the pancreas of one patient who had been taking Januvia. The published report stated,

> since the standard of care of a pancreatic neuroendocrine tumor, because of the risk of conversion to malignancy [cancer], even if benign, is surgical resection [i.e. removal], patients exposed to incretin therapy would seem to be at increased risk of requiring pancreatic surgery.

Pancreatic surgery, even if it doesn't require the removal of your pancreas, is very likely to damage it to the point where you become fully dependent on insulin. And that's if you're lucky. If you aren't, the tumor may turn out not to be benign. Then like almost everyone diagnosed with pancreatic cancer, you will die of it.

The pancreases of the people who had had diabetes but had not taken these drugs displayed none of these abnormal patterns: no cell overgrowth, cells invading the pancreatic ducts, or precancerous glandular tumors.

Upon the publication of Dr. Butler's study, other academic experts hailed it in the pages of the *New York Times* as high quality work. Only drug company flacks were quoted as questioning its validity. But immediately afterward, the drug industry hastened to do major damage control. They pointed out that the people in Dr. Butler's study who had not been taking incretin drugs were largely people with Type 1, suggesting that it was the supposedly gluttonous lifestyle of Type 2s that caused the abnormal cell growth found in their pancreases, not the drugs they were taking—a claim disproven by the Johns Hopkins study.

The drug companies also pointed to a new epidemiological study which, you won't be surprised to learn, showed no additional rates of pancreatitis in users of incretin drugs. But this study did not include people taking either Januvia and Byetta, the incretin drugs with the longest histories of use. It only analyzed statistics derived from people taking Onglyza and Nesina, two much newer incretin drugs with little market penetration.

A more recent study of 14,671 patients given either Januvia or a placebo for three years, undertaken to see if Januvia worsened heart disease was published in 2015. After concluding that Januvia only lowered A1c on average by -0.29% (i.e. from 8% to 7.71%) it concluded that in this population, Januvia taken for three years didn't appear to raise the risk of acute pancreatitis or pancreatic cancer. Though the doctors on Big Pharma's payroll hailed these two studies as proof that these drugs are safe, using their logic you could easily prove that smoking cigarettes is completely safe, too, since it takes far longer than three years for the cancer-producing effects of smoking to emerge.

Before being swayed by drug company arguments, you should note that at the time of their deaths none of the participants in Dr. Butler's autopsy study who were found to have highly abnormal cells in their pancreases had been given a diagnosis of acute pancreatitis or of anything else that would have hinted at problems with their pancreases. The highly abnormal structures growing in their ducts and their small, precancerous glandular tumors were found only on autopsy. It might have taken several more years for those abnormal structures to cause pancreatitis. It might have taken another 10 years or more for those small precancerous tumors to become cancerous and even longer for their cancers to grow large enough to cause the symptoms that would lead to their being diagnosed. But since pancreatic cancer is almost always fatal by the time it is large enough to be diagnosed, by the time these drug-related cancers were detected it would have been too late to save their lives.

Other Serious Side Effects Associated with DPP-4 Inhibitors

The possibility that DPP-4 inhibitors like Januvia may be causing permanent changes in the cells of your pancreas leading to potentially fatal pancreatitis or tumors should be enough to make you skim the rest of this section. But just in case you are still thinking of trying one, there are some other serious side effects associated with inhibiting the DPP-4 gene.

DPP-4 Inhibition Promotes Inflammation

It turns out that apart from regulating blood sugar, DPP-4 also plays an important role in the immune system, where it lowers the level of a proinflammatory peptide, substance P. So inhibiting DPP-4 raises the circulating levels of this inflammatory substance. However, the approval process for Januvia did not require any study of the impact of inhibiting DPP-4 for 24 hours each day on its role in the immune system. An unrelated study, however, that measured the concentrations of DPP-4 in mice with an induced autoimmune arthritis and in humans with rheumatoid arthritis found that the lower the DPP-4 levels, the higher the degree of inflammation.

A helpful email from a leading DPP-4 researcher who sent me some publications about Januvia that are not available on the web, suggests that Januvia is likely to cause more persistent inflammation during the healing of wounds and elsewhere in the body. That's because another function of DPP-4 is to cut up and get rid of cytokines, which are the substances that cause inflammation. So when DPP-4 is inhibited, the cytokines that cause inflammation may rise to higher levels.

This appears to be exactly what happens. Though I had received several reports from people who had developed crippling joint pain after taking Januvia, beginning shortly after its release in 2006, it was only in 2015 that the FDA issued a Safety Announcement, warning that

> The type 2 diabetes medicines sitagliptin [Januvia], saxagliptin [Onglyza], linagliptin [Trajenta] and alogliptin [Nesina] may cause joint pain that can be severe and disabling.

I have also received occasional reports from people who have experienced serious rashes after taking Januvia. The revised Prescribing Information currently warns that it can be linked to a very severe skin condition, Stevens-Johnson Syndrome, in which all a person's skin peels off, leaving them with life altering burns. However, since this condition is extremely rare, doctors are not likely to consider rashes as being caused by the DPP-4 family of drugs.

Inhibiting DPP-4 Turns off Its Ability to Destroy Cancer Genes

As you learned earlier, Januvia and the other DPP-4 inhibitors work by inhibiting the expression of the gene that produces the enzyme that destroys GLP-1. This gene is actually called by various names depending on what kind of scientist is referring to it. When it is destroying GLP-1 it is called DPP-4, sometimes written DPPIV. But cancer researchers call this same gene CD26. And the fact that this drug is of interest not only to endocrinologists but to those studying cancer points to a major concern with this family of drugs. Because the gene they suppress happens to be one that plays an important role in fighting cancer.

It turns out that when you suppress DPP-4 it becomes much easier for melanocytes and prostate cells to transform into malignant cancer cells. As one research study explains, "downregulation of DPPIV [i.e. DPP-4] is an important early event in the pathogenesis of melanoma."

The report continues,

> Malignant cells, including melanomas and carcinomas, frequently lose or alter DPPIV cell surface expression. Loss of DPPIV expression occurs during melanoma progression at a stage where transformed melanocytes become independent of exogenous growth factors for survival. [I.e. the cells stop expressing DPPIV when they start to turn into viable tumor cells.]

More importantly, "Reexpressing DPPIV in melanoma cells at or below levels expressed by normal melanocytes induced a profound change in phenotype that was characteristic of normal melanocytes." In short, turning DPP-4 expression back on stopped the cells from behaving like cancer cells. A similar effect was observed with ovarian cancer cells. The researchers state,

> We investigated the correlation between DPPIV expression and progressive potential in ovarian carcinoma. We demonstrated that ovarian carcinoma *cell lines with higher DPPIV expression were less invasive.* [Emphasis mine]

A study testing the effect of inhibiting DPP-4 in cancerous prostate cells concluded, "By inhibiting CD26/DPPIV, invasion and metastasis of PCa [prostate cancer] cell lines were enhanced in *in vitro* and *in vivo* metastasis assays."

As I'm a melanoma survivor, this information convinced me to stop taking Januvia immediately, despite the fact that it normalized my blood sugars. I cannot afford to play around with any chemical that might be hastening the process by which rogue melanocytes become malignant!

Doesn't FDA Drug Testing Rule Out Drugs that Cause Cancer?

Many people respond to the information you just read by assuming that it is alarmist, because they know that before the FDA approves a drug, it has to pass tests that validate that it doesn't turn normal cells malignant in the lab and that rodents exposed to high levels of the drug don't develop cancers. The DPP-4 inhibitor drugs approved by the FDA obviously must have passed those tests.

But the reason that DPP-4 inhibitors like Januvia may promote cancer isn't that they make normal cells malignant. They don't. Instead, what they may be doing is blocking the mechanism by which the body eliminates cancerous cells once *something else* has made them malignant.

A noted cancer researcher who is an expert on DPP-4's relationship to cancers wrote the following in response to my email asking whether drugs that inhibit DPP-4 posed a cancer threat,

We have shown that loss of DPPIV is indeed associated with melanoma, prostate and lung cancers. Importantly our work has shown that restoring DPPIV can suppress the tumor growth. I have not conducted any detailed studies with DPPIV inhibitors including Januvia, in particular. DPPIV has multiple functions. It is not known if Januvia blocks all of its functions. This warrants more studies with this drug.

So far, no such studies have been done. It is of course true that over time, if these drugs were causing a higher than normal amount of cancer, it should show up in studies of large populations, but because of how slowly cancers grow until they are large enough to be detectible, it can take a decade or more until this kind of signal shows up in epidemiological research, and even then, it won't show up unless scientists are specifically looking for it. Since family doctors are not aware that Januvia may be promoting cancers like melanoma, ovarian cancer, and prostate cancer, they are unlikely to report it to the FDA when a patient who has been taking one of these drugs for many years develops one of these common cancers. So, since The FDA only issues warnings and alerts when it receives a significant number of reports linking a drug to a bad outcome, the connection may remain undiscovered.

Other Common Side Effects of DPP-4 Inhibitors

Less severe but bothersome side effects of DPP-4 inhibitors include sinus headaches and cold symptoms, which may increase in severity and frequency the longer the drug is taken. These too are a result of inhibiting the DPP-4 gene, as it plays yet another role in the sinuses. Then there are a group of side effects that result from the way that high levels of GLP-1 slow digestion: heartburn, delayed stomach emptying, upper abdominal bloating after meals, and constipation.

The DPP-4 Inhibitor Onglyza has Other Serious Side Effects

Onglyza, another DPP-4 inhibitor, has been shown—in the same study used to "prove" that it doesn't cause pancreatitis—to be linked to a higher incidence of heart failure. Onglyza was developed at the same time as Januvia, but its release was long blocked by FDA regulators due to its ability to cause "skin lesions," some of which necrotized [made the skin die and fall off] in monkeys.

Though it was eventually approved, Onglyza offers nothing not offered by Januvia, while the studies cited in the official FDA Prescribing Information for this drug suggest that it has *less* impact on blood sugar than Januvia does while having a *more negative impact* on the immune system's white blood cells. In one person in 100 who take it, Onglyza lowers the white blood count to a dangerously low level.

If your doctor prescribes Onglyza without requiring that you have a periodic CBC blood test, you can be sure the doctor has not read the prescribing information. Few doctors do.

Onglyza also causes some other problems that don't arise with Januvia. For example, because of the way it is metabolized by the liver, Onglyza may build up in the blood stream to unhealthy levels when taken with the yeast medication, ketoconazole, or with other drugs and substances that inhibit specific liver enzymes. These include erythromycin, the calcium channel blocker verapamil, and grapefruit juice. The manufacturer says that the dose of Onglyza must be lowered in people using these drugs. Onglyza levels also rise in people with poorly functioning kidneys. Whether busy doctors will know this and warn patients about lowering the dose when needed is another story.

If Onglyza is prescribed along with Actos or sulfonylurea drugs it raises the peak concentration of these drugs in the bloodstream, which can cause hypos. The icing on this toxic cake is that Onglyza also reduces the peak concentration of metformin.

The Problem with Combining DPP-4 Inhibitors with Metformin

All the DPP-4 inhibitor drugs are also sold in expensive combo pills, which combine the drug with the otherwise cheap generic drug metformin. These include Janumet (Januvia and metformin), Kombiglyze (Onglyza and metformin), and Jentadueto (Trajenta and metformin.) The drug companies love these combinations because metformin is so effective that adding it to their new drugs makes the blood sugar control achieved by the expensive combo pill much more impressive.

Setting aside the concerns we have just looked at concerning the dangerous side effects of these drugs, these pills—and all combo pills—are a poor choice for several other reasons. The most important is that different people need different sized doses of metformin but when the two drugs are combined in one pill you can't increase the size of the metformin dose without increasing the dose of the other drug, which might result in too large a dose of it being given.

The other problem with DPP-4 inhibitor combination pills is that because these drugs slow stomach emptying, the DPP-4 inhibitor can amplify the stomach-related side effects associated with metformin. People who have taken the DPP-4 inhibitors with a separate metformin pill report that they can eliminate stomach discomfort by taking the metformin pill an hour or two *before* the Januvia so that the metformin gets digested before the Januvia shuts down stomach emptying. Taking the two together can result in gas, nausea, and cramps.

Unfortunately, I have heard from several people with Type 2 Diabetes who report that when they experienced stomach problems with Janumet their doctors moved them to plain Januvia—taking them off metformin entirely. This deprived them of the proven cardiovascular and possible anti-cancer benefits of metformin, as well as of its ability to lower insulin resistance. They were left with only the very expensive DPP-4 inhibitor that does nothing but slightly increase their insulin secretion, while exposing them to all the dangers we have cited.

GLP-1 Agonists also Have Other Severe Side Effects

Though the problems with the DPP-4 inhibitor pills are best known, given how widely they have been prescribed, other problems are also emerging with drugs in the injected GLP-1 receptor agonist class.

They May Be Dangerous for People with Damaged Kidneys

In late 2009 the FDA analyzed postmarketing data for Byetta and found 78 cases of kidney failure reported between April 28, 2005 and October 29, 2008, a period in which more than 6.6 million prescriptions for Byetta had been dispensed. The FDA-approved Prescribing Information for Byetta and Bydureon now warns that they "should not be used in patients with severe renal [i.e. kidney] impairment" and that "caution should be applied when initiating" them or when raising the dose in patients "with moderate renal impairment." In earlier versions of this label the FDA defined "severe renal impairment" as "creatinine clearance <30 ml/min" and "moderate renal impairment as "creatinine clearance 30 to 50 ml/min)."

Check your creatinine clearance before you take any of these drugs. Your creatinine clearance should appear on the annual labs your doctor should be doing. Make sure your doctor gives you a copy of the actual test results, not just the reassurance that "everything was fine." When you get the actual report, you may find that your doctor's idea of "fine" includes not only an A1c well over 7% but a creatinine clearance value pointing to moderate renal impairment. This is because doctors often expect people with diabetes to have deteriorating kidney function.

Victoza does not carry this warning, however, the official prescribing information states,

> There is limited experience in patients with mild, moderate, and severe renal impairment, including end-stage renal disease. Therefore, Victoza should be used with caution in this patient population.

It is quite possible that similar problems with Victoza will emerge once as many people have taken it as have taken the older drug, Byetta.

Thyroid Cancer

Because it only needs to be injected once rather than twice a day, Victoza is now the bestselling GLP-1 receptor agonist drug, taking Byetta's place. However the FDA-mandated Prescribing Information for Victoza suggests that its side effect profile is even more troubling than that of Byetta, while its impact on blood sugars is less impressive. Concerns about those side effects were such that the FDA delayed its approval for several years. When it was finally released, Victoza's official prescribing information carried a black box warning stating that it may produce thyroid cancers. It still does.

Though its maker claims this should only be a problem in rodents, the European prescribing information for Victoza, which was available on the web before Victoza was approved in the United States, revealed that human trials had shown that, "in liraglutide [Victoza]-treated patients, thyroid neoplasms [i.e. cancers] ... were reported in 0.5% ... of patients ." The control group had none.

If you are taking Liraglutide for weight loss, in the form of Saxenda, be aware that the dose is higher than the dose used in the diabetes clinical trials, which may raise these risks.

Less Serious but Significant Side Effects of GLP-1 Agonists

Because GLP-1 receptor agonists cause the valve at the bottom of your stomach to close, they can produce severe nausea and even vomiting. Other side effects that have been reported anecdotally online are tooth pain, and a persistent feeling of cold.

Safety Concerns Should Keep You From Trying These Drugs

Those of you who read the earlier edition of this book know that, like so many others, I was misled by the attempts of the drug makers to debunk the epidemiological research linking Byetta to pancreatitis, and hence recommended that people with diabetes try it because it had been reported to be so very effective in about one third of the people who tried it.

But after reading Dr. Butler's autopsy research study and his subsequent review of the many other studies that hinted that these drugs were causing abnormal patterns of cell growth in the pancreas I have concluded that they are too dangerous to experiment with.

The cellular changes these drugs appear to make to cells and structures in the pancreases of rodents and of the people Dr. Butler autopsied are permanent. They occur long before any symptoms of pancreatitis become evident.

The drug makers do currently warn doctors that pancreatitis may be a risk with these drugs—they must, because the FDA forces them to do so—but they continue to state that the remedy for this is that doctors should take patients off these drugs at the first sign of symptoms. But this won't help. By the time pancreatitis causes symptoms, abnormal cells will have already grown throughout the pancreas. For most patients experiencing the intense pain, nausea or swiftly rising blood sugars characteristic of pancreatitis, it will be too late to undo the damage the drugs have already done.

This makes these drugs far too dangerous to mess with. The benefits they produce in most people are too limited to justify the risk they present.

SGLT2 Inhibitors: Drugs that Alter Kidney Function

The SGLT2 inhibitors are a new family of drugs that use a novel mechanism to lower blood sugar. While other drugs remove glucose from the blood by boosting insulin levels or reducing insulin resistance, these drugs do it by changing how your kidneys function, so that they excrete more glucose via urine.

Normally, your kidneys won't extract glucose from your blood and excrete it until your blood sugar reaches a certain threshold that lies somewhere between 160 and 180 mg/dl. The exact threshold varies from person to person, and in some individuals it can be much higher. But these new SGLT-2 drugs lower that threshold so that your kidneys excrete far more glucose—100 grams a day according to the official Prescribing Information for one of these drugs, Invokana. Since peeing away 100 grams of glucose will also dispose of 400 calories that would otherwise turn into fat, these drugs are also capable of causing weight loss.

Invokana (generic name, canagliflozin), was the first drug in this family to be approved for sale in the United States, back in 2013. It is also found in Invokamet, a combo pill that also contains metformin. Invokana quickly became a "blockbuster" drug, selling over a billion dollars worth in a single year.

Next to be approved was Farxiga, mysteriously named "Forxiga" outside of the United States. Both drugs are generically named dapagliflozin. Dapagliflozin is also sold as Xigduo, a combination pill containing Farxiga and metformin.

Jardiance is the latest drug in this family to have been approved. Its generic name is empagliflozin. Not only is Jardiance sold in a combo pill where it is combined with metformin, marketed under the name Synjardy, but it is also found in a different combo pill, Glyxambi, where it is combined with the DPP-4 inhibitor Trajenta.

Other drug companies are currently working on getting approval for yet more members of this new drug family.

Side Effects According to the Official Prescribing Information

Yeast and Urinary Tract Infections

These drugs can cause serious yeast infections in women and uncircumcised men. This is no surprise, as yeast thrive in a damp, sugary environment. That's why frequent yeast infections are often the first symptom of undiagnosed diabetes.

One in ten people who took Invokana experienced yeast infections. In addition, one in twenty who took it experienced bladder and other urinary tract infections. These kinds of infections are a side effect of all drugs in the SGLT2 Inhibitor family.

Decreased Kidney Function

This too is a class effect applying to all drugs in the SGLT-2 inhibitor family. The Prescribing Information for Invokana states: "INVOKANA increases serum creatinine and decreases eGFR [glomerular filtration rate.]" Drugs in this family also raise the risk of dehydration, dangerous low blood pressure, and hyperalkemia (high potassium levels), especially in people taking blood pressure medication. Untreated, hyperalkemia can lead to heart rhythm abnormalities, which in some cases can be fatal. Older people, particularly those over 75, are those most likely to experience the most severe kidney-based side effects from these drugs.

Low Blood Pressure and Dizziness

Because these drugs make people urinate far more frequently than usual, they can cause low blood pressure and severe dizziness. These effects are more likely to occur in people with compromised kidney function or in the elderly.

Hypoglycemia in People Taking Insulin or Insulin Stimulating Drugs

These drugs must be used cautiously if you are injecting insulin or taking an insulin stimulating drug of any kind—sulfonylureas, meglitinides, or even, possibly, incretin drugs, to avoid hypos. The Prescribing Information for these drugs warns that doses of insulin and insulin-stimulating drugs should be lowered if these drugs are being taken.

Increased "Bad" Cholesterol

All these drugs list elevated LDL-C as a known side effect in their official Prescribing Information.

Raised Cancer Risk

The prescribing information for Farxiga notes that an "imbalance" in cases of bladder cancer was found in the clinical trials for this drug.

This was not observed in trials for the other SGLT2 inhibitor drugs, but given how new they are, and how long cancers take to develop, the possibility that this is a class effect should not be ignored. At a minimum, it should be remembered that glucose is the favorite food of tumors, so the high glucose levels that these drugs cause in the organs of the urinary tract may promote the growth of any previously undetected cancers that may be silently growing in them.

The FDA eventually approved Farxiga but is mandating a post-marketing study to verify that these drugs do not cause bladder cancer. Unfortunately, thousands of people will take the drug during the period of several years before the results of this study is available.

The side effects listed above are the ones that showed up during the clinical trials that were run as part of the drug approval process. As we've have seen with the other drugs we've discussed, these trials rarely discover all the serious side effects of any drug, since it is only after tens or hundreds of thousands of people have taken them for many years that their real side effects can be detected.

User Experience with SGLT2 Inhibitors Is Mixed

Posts in online communities suggest that these drugs work very well for some people, including some with Type 1 Diabetes who take them off-label and find that they lower the amount of insulin they need to inject. Some people also are reporting that they experience welcome weight loss while they take them.

However, others report that these drugs make them feel ill. In many cases this seems to be because the greatly increased urination they cause leads to dehydration, even when people increase their water intake. This is because excess urination can easily deplete electrolytes.

The yeast infections mentioned in the Prescribing Information don't affect everyone, but when they do, they can be problematic. Some women report that they have developed nasty, drug resistant yeast infections while taking one of these drugs. These were hard to eradicate even after they discontinued the drug.

FDA Safety Alerts Point to More Serious Side Effects

Ketoacidosis in People with Type 2 Diabetes

The FDA issued a warning on May 15, 2015 stating that it had received a significant number of aftermarket reports linking this family of drugs to ketoacidosis. **Ketoacidosis** is a very serious, potentially fatal condition where the levels of ketones and acid in the blood rise dangerously high. Ketoacidosis makes people very sick and if untreated can be fatal. Symptoms of ketoacidosis include: difficulty breathing, nausea, vomiting, abdominal pain, confusion, and unusual fatigue or sleepiness. It requires a trip to the emergency room.

What is particularly worrisome here is that ketoacidosis usually *only* occurs in people with Type 1 diabetes, and then only when they have extremely high blood sugars. However, in the cases reported to the FDA, ketoacidosis was occurring in people with Type 2 Diabetes who had only modestly elevated blood sugars. This makes it likely that the SGLT2 drugs are causing ketoacidosis by preventing the kidneys from eliminate ketones from the bloodstream as they build, up the way kidneys normally do.

This might pose a danger to people eating diets very low in carbohydrates who often have higher than normal ketone levels in their blood. When kidneys are functioning normally, this is perfectly safe, as long as blood sugars are not extremely high. But those high ketone levels may *not* be benign for people taking SGLT2 inhibitors, since it is possible that even at near normal blood sugar levels these drugs may block the normal processes the kidneys use to keep ketone levels within a safe range.

Until we have a much better understanding of exactly what it is that is leading to ketoacidosis in people taking the SGLT2 inhibitor drugs, you should *not* take them while eating a very low carb diet. For most people, a low carb diet starts raising blood ketone levels when their daily carbohydrate intake drops below 110 g a day.

Bone Fracture Risk and Decreased Bone Mineral Density

On Sept 10, 2015, the FDA issued a Safety Alert for Invokana and Invokamet, stating that,

> Bone fractures have been seen in patients taking the type 2 diabetes medicine canagliflozin [Invokana]. Fractures can occur as early as 12 weeks after starting canagliflozin. Canagliflozin has also been linked to decreases in bone mineral density at the hip and lower spine.

Though the warning specifically mentioned Invokana, the oldest drug in this family, the warning bulletin also said,

> FDA is continuing to evaluate the risk of bone fractures with other drugs in the SGLT2 inhibitor class, including dapagliflozin (Farxiga, Xigduo XR) and empaglifozin (Jardiance, Glyxambi, Synjardy), to determine if additional label changes or studies are needed.

This side effect probably occurs because messing with how the kidneys excrete glucose also affects how they handle the minerals used build bones: phosphorus, calcium, and magnesium. Note that once your bones have become weakened, it can become difficult or even impossible to rebuild them. This, along with the fact that these drugs are more likely to cause severe dizziness in people over 65, suggests that older people in particular should avoid these drugs. The elderly are already at higher risk for osteoporosis, and dizziness raises the likelihood of falls which can lead to fractures.

Anyone who has taken either Avandia or Actos for any significant period of time should also avoid these new drugs, as those drugs were also found to cause bone thinning, not all of which is detectible using the usual tests used to screen for osteoporosis.

If your doctor prescribes one of these drugs, ask if they are aware of these two recent FDA safety warnings. Chances are that they may have missed them.

Research Claims Jardiance Cuts Cardiovascular Risk

There was excitement in the medical community after a study was published in the *New England Journal of Medicine* in September of 2015, which was reported by the media as showing that people with Type 2 Diabetes who were taking Jardiance had a 38% lower risk of cardiovascular death.

This was blockbuster news, as no other patented drug for Type 2 Diabetes can make this claim. As we have seen earlier, the risk for heart disease rises dramatically as A1cs near 7%, even though this is the level most doctors tell their patients to strive for. So we can expect that a huge marketing budget will be devoted to getting doctors to prescribe this drug to all their patients with Type 2 Diabetes.

But closer inspection of the actual published study, makes it clear that the drug company press releases that were sent to the media exaggerated the actual findings. For example, the researchers in this study only gave the drug to people with Type 2 Diabetes who had *already* had a heart attack, stroke, stenting, unstable angina, or a failed stress test—people who were already quite ill with heart disease. Though some of them did do better on the drug, this provides no evidence that Jardiance would be equally effective in people with Type 2 Diabetes whose better blood sugar control has kept them free of heart disease.

And the "38% risk reduction" cited in the press release grossly inflates the actual impact of the drug. This is because "risk reduction" is a statistical trick that is used to turn a very small statistical difference into a larger one. For example, if three people out of one thousand have a heart attack, and a drug reduces that number to only two people out of a thousand, the drug has reduced the "*risk*" of a heart attack by 33%—as one is 33% of three. But the actual rate at which heart attacks occurred in the population has only decreased from .3% to .2%.

And in fact, the numbers published in the study show that Jardiance reduced the incidence of any serious cardiovascular event by about 1.5% in the group as a whole. Over the course of the study 10.5% of the people taking Jardiance who had already experienced a serious cardiovascular event had another one, compared to 12.1% of those in the placebo group. This made a difference of only 1.6% in the actual number of events that occurred—one and a half fewer events per 100 people. This is much less impressive sounding than that original 38% "risk" reduction.

A table published separately in a Supplemental Appendix to the study shows that although the total number of all cardiovascular events was, indeed, lower among the entire group of people who took Jardiance, when the researchers split out subgroups of people, they found that slightly *more* people had fatal and nonfatal strokes in the group taking Jardiance than in the group taking the placebo. More people taking Jardiance also had a specific kind of heart attack, a silent myocardial infarction, on Jardiance than did those in the placebo group. More people were hospitalized for unstable angina in the group taking a lower dose of Jardiance than in the placebo group.

Subgroup analysis also showed that Blacks, people with better kidney function, people with A1cs over 8.5%, people with peripheral artery disease, and people using insulin did *better* in terms of avoiding cardiovascular events when taking a placebo than those taking Jardiance. People over 65 did very slightly better on placebo, too.

The bottom line seems to be that if you have serious heart disease and take this drug, your chance of having a heart attack or heart failure goes down slightly, while your chance of having a fatal or nonfatal stroke goes up very slightly. This probably is because the excess urination caused by SGLT2 drugs lowers both blood volume and blood pressure through its dehydrating effect. But this study produced no evidence at all that this drug will prevent the development of heart disease in people with Type 2 Diabetes who don't already have it.

Jardiance Did a Poor Job Lowering Blood Sugar

In fact, taking Jardiance in place of a more effective drug might actually *raise* the likelihood of developing heart disease. That's because this study also found that Jardiance did a very poor job of lowering the A1cs of those who took it. The starting A1cs of the people in this study ranged from 7% to 10%. But after the people taking Jardiance had taken the drug for 94 weeks, their average A1c had only dropped 0.47% when compared to that of the people taking a placebo. So those who started with A1cs of 10% may still have had A1cs as high as 9.53%.

As time went on, their response to the drug got worse. By week 206, the difference in the average A1c between those taking Jardiance and those taking placebo was only 0.36%. By the end of the study, the average A1c of those taking Jardiance was 7.81%. As this is an average, it implies that a lot of people on this drug still had A1cs well above 8%. That means they still had a greatly increased risk of developing heart disease. And that's not all. Living with an A1c near 8% is also likely to damage the kidneys, though as we just saw, further kidney damage is already a known concern with this family of drugs.

Diet, exercise, metformin, and if needed, properly prescribed insulin, are all much more likely to lower your blood sugar to a safer, heart and kidney protecting level than is Jardiance.

There Is No Compelling Reason to Take SGLT2 Inhibitors Now

Though I risk sounding like a broken record, once again it seems clear that the risks outweigh the benefits when it comes to taking these new, heavily marketed drugs whose true side effects won't be understood for a decade or more. Drug companies have too much incentive to hype their most profitable drugs and to inflate the findings of the research they pay for. This hype is always strongest when their drugs have only been available for two or three years, as is the case with all the new SGLT2 inhibitors.

No one really knows what the long-term impact will be of changing the way that your kidneys work, and given that kidneys are already under stress in most people with diabetes, there is little reason to become one of the guinea pigs used to find out.

How Can You Stay Safe with New Drugs?

After reading the above you may be wondering if it is safe to take *any* new drug. The answer is a qualified "maybe." Because it takes at least a decade for the real side effects of any new drug to become known, you have to be very cautious when weighing the benefits claimed for new drugs against their hidden risks you can't possibly know about.

Be skeptical about any new drug unless it cures a condition that, left untreated, will shorten your life or leave you with symptoms worse than any likely side effects. A new drug that halts fatal cancer or one that has a good chance of keeping you from going blind would be worth taking. A new drug that lowers A1c by .49% is another story. Here are a few guidelines to keep you safe:

❖ Before you take *any* new drug, download the PDF containing the official Prescribing Information for that drug, which you can find on the manufacturer's web site. The "Prescribing Information" is the "label" required by the FDA. It has to be kept up-to-date. Your pharmacist can also give you copies of the latest version of the

Prescribing Information.

❖ The Prescribing Information will list all the known serious side effects of a drug. Even though the FDA usually allows a drug to stay on the market when a serious side effect is discovered, it does make the drug company mention the side effect in the Prescribing Information. The Prescribing Information will also mention whether these drugs may pose special dangers for older people, people with specific medical conditions, or people taking other drugs.

❖ Make sure you understand the Prescribing Information. If your medical knowledge isn't good enough to understand the wording, don't be shy about calling up your doctor's office and asking someone there to interpret it for you. The information contained in the Prescribing Information may be as big a surprise to your doctor as it is to you. If you are concerned about a possible drug interaction, contact a registered pharmacist at the pharmacy where you got the drug and ask if you should stop taking the drug. Pharmacists are often better informed about drug safety than are busy doctors.

❖ If a drug can produce serious side effects, ask your doctor whether there are tests that can spot these side effects early enough to prevent permanent damage. Then make sure your doctor does those tests. Even then, there is still the concern that the drug company may have told your doctor that certain tests can guarantee safety when this is not true. With the failed TZD drug Rezulin, the drug company advised doctors to test liver enzymes. But by the time liver enzyme tests warned of liver damage, it was too late to reverse the damage for some of the victims who died of liver failure.

❖ Ask your doctor if there is an older, better understood drug that could be used instead of the newer drug.

❖ If your doctor claims that a new drug does something really important that no other drug does, such as grow new beta cells, prevent heart attacks, or heal diabetic complications, check out the actual research backing up this claim. You can usually find it discussed on the **bloodsugar101.com** web site.

All this sounds like a lot of work, and it is. But since your doctor is too busy to do it, you will have to. It's *your* body that will pay the price if you take a toxic drug.

Chapter Ten
Insulin

Nothing raises as much fear in the minds of most people with Type 2 Diabetes as the thought of having to go on insulin. This is a tragedy, because, of all the medications available to diabetics, insulin is the only one capable of not just lowering, but of normalizing, their blood sugar.

There are lots of things about diabetes that should be terrifying, like impotence, blindness, amputation, kidney failure, and, worst of all, the very high likelihood of dying, much too young, of a heart attack. All these are caused by prolonged exposure to high blood sugars, including blood sugars reaching levels that many doctors consider too low to be worthy of any drug treatment at all. Since insulin can prevent all these terrible things from happening, why waste your fear on it?

We'll look now at what people with diabetes fear about insulin and examine why their fears are groundless.

Needles

Needles scare a lot of us because the needles used to give immunization shots and draw blood hurt. Fortunately, insulin needles are much thinner and don't. It comes as a pleasant surprise to many people with Type 2 Diabetes to discover that the ultra-thin, very short needles used for injecting insulin are even less painful than the lancets they use to test their blood sugar. Most of the time these needles are so painless that when you inject you may have to take a close look to see if you have actually penetrated the skin, because you can't feel the needle.

Insulin is injected into the layer of fat that lies just under the skin, so insulin needles can be almost as thin as hairs. They don't need to penetrate tough muscles or enter blood vessels the way immunization and blood drawing needles do. However, some older family doctors may be unaware that very thin, very short insulin needles are available now and may instead prescribe old-fashioned, long, thick needles. Those *can* be painful. If you were first prescribed insulin at a hospital, you probably were given shots with a long, thick needle. The reason for this is that there is always the possibility that the hospital staff members who give injections might be exposed to blood borne diseases. So hospitals mandate that staff use specially capped needles that have been designed to make it less likely they will stick themselves. These needles only come in thicker gauges.

But blood borne disease is not a problem for you when you are injecting yourself, so insist that your doctor prescribe the thinnest, shortest needle possible. Ask a pharmacist to recommend the best needle for you, if your doctor doesn't have up-to-date information about needle gauges. Research has found even very heavy people can use the very short 5 mm needles, which some doctors don't yet know.

The second important thing to know about injecting insulin is that when you first start out and are panicking at the idea of giving yourself a shot, you can just pinch up a thick fold of tummy fat and "throw" the syringe at the fat the way you'd throw a dart, holding the syringe tightly with three fingers and tossing it at your target, starting from 6 or 7 inches away. The swift motion of the needle eliminates any sting or feeling of the needle going in and will help you get over your natural anxiety about injecting yourself. Once you are used to injecting, all you have to do is just push the needle into a pinch of fat.

If your insurance will cover insulin pens, they are much easier to use than insulin supplied in a vial and injected with a syringe, especially if you need to use insulin at work or at a restaurant. Pens containing insulin let you select the exact number of units you want to inject and then press a button to dispense it.

You will still need a separate prescription for the pen needles that are screwed into the tip of the "pen" that holds the insulin. So again, it is important to make sure you are prescribed the most appropriately sized needles.

Fear of Hypos

The other major fear that keeps people with Type 2 Diabetes from using insulin is the fear that they will have dangerous or even fatal hypo after taking too much insulin. We've all seen the movies where someone goes into "insulin shock" and nearly dies. This fear also keeps doctors from prescribing insulin to people with Type 2 Diabetes.

Hypos are a possibility, but a 2010 study found that patients using insulin had *fewer* hypos then patients taking Actos or the sulfonylurea drug glyburide. The advantage of injecting insulin is that you have a lot more control over the *dose* of insulin you get than you do with an insulin-stimulating pill. So if you take some time to study how to use insulin you should be able to avoid serious hypos completely.

And make no mistake: using insulin safely does take some study. It's more work than swallowing a pill. But unlike most pills, insulin works. If you learn how to get the dosing right and keep your carbohydrates under control, insulin can lower any blood sugar to a safe and normal level.

Fear of Weight Gain

Many patients—and their doctors—also fear that injecting insulin will lead to weight gain. However, the study cited in the previous section also found that patients using insulin experienced *less* weight gain than those taking Actos or glyburide.

Fear that Insulin Raises Heart Disease Risk

Because published research shows that people with diabetes using injected insulin are more likely to have heart attacks than those not using it, many doctors have assumed that it is the insulin causing these heart attacks. This is wrong. The only reason that insulin use is associated with excess heart attacks is that for decades most doctors have delayed prescribing insulin to patients with Type 2 Diabetes until they have spent many years living with the extremely high blood sugars that are the real cause of those heart attacks. Many doctors won't insist a patient go on insulin until their A1c has been above 9% or 10% for years. As we noted in Chapter Four, the risk of heart attack doubles for every 1% rise in A1c over 4.6%. So these years of exposure to uncontrolled very high blood sugars damage the arteries, sometimes irreversibly. This is what makes so many people with Type 2 Diabetes more prone to heart attacks at the time they are finally put on insulin.

Another factor that has linked insulin use to heart problems is that for years doctors were not informed by the drug companies that people who take insulin along with Actos and Avandia are more likely to experience heart failure. Fortunately, this is now known and these drugs are much less commonly prescribed with insulin.

But there is no evidence that people who begin insulin use before they have suffered those years of poor control and who use it to achieve normal blood sugars share this same risk.

The FDA has forced drug companies to test all their new, patented insulins to ensure that they do not, on their own, raise the risk of heart disease. All the new insulins have passed these tests.

Once on Insulin Always on Insulin?

Another reason people fear insulin is that they may have heard that once you start insulin you will never be able to stop using it. Observing what happened to their diabetic relatives, they may also conclude that once a person starts insulin it is only a matter of time until they suffer blindness, amputation, and kidney failure.

This misunderstanding is also caused by the fact that in the past many doctors delayed giving patients insulin until long after they needed it. So by the time patients started it, they were contending with decades of damage produced by exposure to very high blood sugars.

Up-to-date doctors now know that if they intervene early and use insulin to bring down extremely high blood sugars soon after diagnosis, people with Type 2 Diabetes are more likely to regain excellent control and be able to stop using insulin. Very high blood sugars greatly increase insulin resistance and using insulin to lower them can improve it. I went off insulin after using it for five years and have better blood sugars now than I did ten years ago.

Insulin Must be Tailored to Your Own Metabolism

The most important thing to understand about insulin is that the dose that works for you is going to be different from the dose that works for someone else, because your physiologies are different. Because of this, when you first start using insulin your doctor should put you on a low dose and ask you to record your blood sugars. Then he should slowly raise the dose in small increments until your blood sugars reach your target levels. If your doctor isn't willing to work with you to pick a starting dose and then work toward adjusting it so that your blood sugars become normal, or refer you to a Certified Diabetes Educator who can help you with this, you probably need to find a better doctor.

Unfortunately, doctors often give people with Type 2 Diabetes generic doses of insulin. If the dose is too high the patient will have to eat a lot of carbohydrate to keep from having hypos. Using a lot of insulin to cover a lot of carbohydrate usually results in the rollercoaster blood sugars we described earlier that cause hunger, overeating, and weight gain. If the generic dose is too small, blood sugars drop only a little bit and remain high enough to damage health, and because blood sugars are still surging and dropping, you may also become very hungry and gain weight.

Because doctors are more concerned that too much insulin may cause hypos than they are about blood sugars that remain dangerously high, many people with Type 2 Diabetes who are prescribed insulin are not given nearly enough insulin to bring their blood sugars down to a safe level. If you are "on insulin" and still routinely seeing blood sugars that are rising well above 200 mg/dl after meals or that remain over 125 mg/dl when you test first thing in the morning, your insulin doses need to be adjusted.

Only when your doctor or educator takes the time to teach you how to adjust your blood sugars so you can "walk up" to the correct dose will you end up with the kind of blood sugars you want. When you have found that right dose, your blood sugars should stay relatively flat and you should not be hungry.

It goes beyond the scope of this book to explain insulin dosing to you in detail, but you can learn what you need to know from a Certified Diabetes Educator (CDE) or a good doctor. Supplement that with what you read in the books *Dr. Bernstein's Diabetes Solution*, by Dr. Richard K. Bernstein or *Think Like a Pancreas*, by Gary Scheiner. *Using Insulin* by John Walsh is another book that is often recommended.

Understanding the Different Kinds of Insulin Available

If you are considering using insulin, it is important to understand that there are quite a few different kinds of insulin that can be prescribed, each with different properties.

First off, all insulins currently available fall into one of two classes: those whose molecules are identical to the insulin your pancreas makes and those whose molecules have been altered in very small ways to change their properties. Insulins in both of these two classes then fall into two more categories: those that replace the slow but steady drip of basal insulin, which lowers fasting blood sugar and those that replace the larger surges of insulin that a normal pancreas secretes at mealtimes. Now let's look more closely at the various kinds of insulin that are available to help you regain normal blood sugars.

Regular Human Insulin

Until the 1980s the insulin given to people with diabetes was extracted from the pancreases of pigs or cows slaughtered for meat. These insulins contained impurities, and there was always the possibility that they could transmit viruses or mad cow disease. But all insulins sold now are artificially produced by bacteria grown in fermentation tanks. These bacteria have been genetically modified to produce the many insulins now on the market.

The insulin called **regular human insulin** (R) was the first lab-created insulin. It was released back in the 1980s. Though it is artificially produced, the regular human insulin molecule itself is identical to the insulin secreted by a human pancreas. It is not patented and can sometimes be bought far more cheaply than the newer, patented insulins.

Novolin, Humulin, and Insuman are brand names under which regular human insulin is sold. The other insulins made with regular human insulin are the NPH insulins sold under the brand names Novolin N and Humulin N. However, the human insulin in these N insulins is not identical to the insulin your pancreas makes as it has been combined with protamine and zinc to slow it down and turn it into a longer-acting insulin. Both the R and N forms of regular human insulin are sold by Walmart pharmacies under the Relion brand name.

Regular Human Insulin is Slow

When your pancreas secretes a human insulin molecule, it releases it directly into the portal vein where it acts very quickly. But when these same human insulin molecules must be absorbed from the fat of an injection site, they can be very slow to take effect.

Because of this, regular human insulin must be injected an hour before a meal if it is to match up properly with the carbohydrates contained in the food. This makes it impossible to eat spontaneously when injecting this kind of insulin, as you must know exactly what you are going to eat an hour ahead of time. If something occurs to keep you from eating a meal after you have injected a dose of regular human insulin to cover it, a serious hypo can occur.

Regular human insulin also lasts a long time. It stays active for five to seven hours or even longer, depending on how much has been injected. This long period of activity raises the risk that the insulin may cause a hypo if it is still being absorbed into the bloodstream long after glucose has stopped coming in from a digested meal.

Analog Insulins

The slowness and long activity curve of regular human insulin made it challenging for people with diabetes to control their blood sugar with it. So when scientists became more familiar with recombinant DNA technology, they were able to develop new insulins whose structures have been slightly modified to alter their properties. These are called **analog insulins**. They are not identical to the insulin your pancreas makes. Instead, they consist of genetically engineered molecules that are very similar to human insulin except that have had one or more amino acids substituted for those found in the naturally occurring human insulin molecule. These very small changes in the structure of the insulin molecule change the speed with which it is absorbed.

Many of us find that we do much better on one particular analog insulin than we do on others of the same class. So if you have trouble lowering your fasting insulin without experiencing hypos when using one type of analog insulin, ask your doctor if you can try a different one. By the same token, if you can't cover mealtime carbs without experiencing spikes or hypos using one brand of analog insulin, ask your doctor to prescribe a different one. As is so often the case with everything involving diabetes, there are significant differences in how individuals respond to specific brands of analog insulin.

Unfortunately, as the prices of analog insulins have doubled over the past decade, many insurance plans only cover the analog insulins made by whichever company has given them the best price discount. If yours does this, you may be stuck having to use the one brand of insulin they cover, even though it isn't the one that would give you the best control. Sometimes your doctor can write a letter to your insurer explaining why you need to use a different kind of insulin and convince your insurer to cover it, even if it is not officially covered. If you are covered by a Medicare drug plan, take a close look at which insulins are covered by any plan you are considering before you sign on.

You will need a prescription to buy any analog insulin, but in most states in the United States you can buy regular human insulin without a prescription, although you may need a prescription for the needles used to inject it. If you are having trouble paying for insulin, it is helpful to know that Walmart usually sells regular human insulin in both the shorter and longer-acting forms for about $29 a vial, which is far cheaper than any other insulin available at other pharmacies.

Though regular human insulin is harder to use if you are trying to cover typical meals containing thirty grams of carbohydrate or more, it can work well in low doses for people who are still seeing high blood sugars after eating meals that are low in carbohydrate.

Biosimilar Insulins

A new class of insulins called **biosimilar insulins** is entering the marketplace now that the patents for many of the original analog insulins are expiring. "Biosimilar" is the term used for a generic version of a substance like insulin that is a protein that must be manufactured using genetically engineered bacteria or fungi.

The FDA and other regulating bodies are supposed to ensure that biosimilars drugs have molecular structures and properties very similar to those of the once-patented drugs they have previously approved.

Some biosimilars are also described as **bioidentical**. This means that the protein they are made of is identical to the patented hormone they replace. There is some question as to whether some of the new biosimilars currently approved for use in Europe are as effective as the patented basal insulins that they emulate. But as long as they are cheaper, insurers will probably force people with diabetes to use these new biosimilars because of the cost savings.

Fast and Slow Insulins

Remember how back in Chapter One we explained that your body secretes insulin in three different phases, basal, first-phase, and second-phase insulin? Well, the kinds of insulin your doctor can prescribe fall into similar categories.

Basal Insulin

Basal insulin attempts to mimic the basal insulin secretion we discussed in Chapter One, which, when it is working properly keeps fasting blood sugar in a narrow range somewhere between 70 and 90 mg/dl. Once injected, basal insulin is very slowly absorbed into the body over a period of several hours. Two or three hours after it has been injected, the level of basal insulin in the bloodstream should level out and provide a steady background dose of insulin. The effect of a single injection of Lantus, the bestselling basal insulin, usually lasts from 18-24 hours. (Lantus' generic name is insulin glargine.) An injection of Levemir (insulin detemir) lasts 12 hours when it is used in the small doses prescribed to people with Type 1 Diabetes, but it may last much longer when administered in the much larger doses prescribed for people with Type 2. Both basal insulins provide a steady dribble of insulin into your bloodstream during the period during which they are active.

Two new patented basal insulins were approved for use in the United States in 2015, around the time that the patent for Lantus expired. Toujeo is made of the same insulin glargine molecule found in Lantus, though in Toujeo that molecule is dissolved in less fluid. This makes it more concentrated, which may have some benefit for people who require very large doses of basal insulin. Otherwise, it is very similar to Lantus.

Tresiba (Insulin Degludec), the other new basal insulin, is a very long-acting basal insulin that is sold by the same company that makes Levemir. Tresiba remains active for up to 42 hours, though its effect starts to wane after 24 hours, so it still needs to be injected once a day to get the most consistent coverage.

Both of these new patented insulins are even more expensive than the ones they replaced and cynics assume, probably correctly, that their real reason for existing is to extend patent protection for their manufacturers. So far, based on the research included with their FDA approved Prescribing Information, there is no evidence that either of these new basal insulins provides any significant advantages over the older insulins, though European authorities, unlike the FDA, have allowed the makers of these insulins to claim that they cause fewer nighttime hypos. If you are doing well using Lantus or Levemir there appears to be no compelling reason to switch to these more expensive basal insulins.

Now that these older insulins have gone off patent, biosimilar versions of insulin glargine will be coming to the market in the United States in 2017. This is the insulin found in Lantus and Toujeo. Some biosimilar basal insulins are already available in Europe. It is expected that the Lantus biosimilars will be priced slightly more cheaply than the patented and formerly patented basal insulins.

NPH

NPH (Humulin N, Novolin N, generic name isophane insulin) is an older, sometimes cheaper, longer-acting insulin. It is made out of Regular Human insulin with zinc and protamine added to slow down its absorption and activity. Though NPH is technically not a basal insulin—it must be injected two or three times a day—it is sometimes prescribed in the place of basal insulin to people with poor or nonexistent health insurance. That is because it can be purchased for far less than the true basal insulins.

NPH does not remain active as long as the newer, patented basal insulins nor does it deliver the relatively stable, flat blood sugars they do, since its concentration in the bloodstream peaks sharply and unpredictably some time between three and thirteen hours after it has been injected. The time and intensity of the peak a person may experience can differ from day to day. This unpredictable activity also makes NPH far more likely to cause hypos than the patented insulins.

Unlike all the other insulins currently on the market, NPH is cloudy. This is because it contains tiny particles. You must gently roll a vial of NPH to mix it before you draw it into a syringe.

Basal Insulin Can't Bring Down High Post-Meal Blood Sugars

It is essential to understand that *no basal insulin can bring down the blood sugar spikes caused by the carbohydrates you eat at meals.* When dosed properly, basal insulin should only lower your fasting and pre-meal blood sugars. If you raise the dose of a basal insulin high enough to counteract a high spike caused by a meal, you are likely to experience a hypo after any prolonged period when you haven't eaten. With longer-acting insulins like Lantus and Tresiba, a dose high enough to completely control blood sugar after high carb meals almost guarantees that you will experience potentially dangerous hypos late at night.

But by now you understand that high blood sugars after meals are the major cause of organ damage. And knowing that, you should be able to see what the problem might be with using an insulin regimen that only involves basal insulin: It can't lower post-meal spikes. This is why so many people with Type 2 Diabetes who are "on insulin" still have A1cs over 7.0%—often way over 7.0%.

Fast-Acting Insulin

Fast-acting insulin is injected to cover a specific meal. The speed of fast-acting insulins varies from product to product, with some being much faster than others. But all the analog fast-acting insulins currently available mimic the normal person's second-phase insulin response we described in Chapter One. These insulins peak in the bloodstream between one and two hours after they are injected and stay active for a total of three to five hours. The fast-acting insulins currently available include Novolog, known as NovoRapid in the UK (generic name, insulin aspart), Humalog (insulin lispro), and Apidra (insulin glulisine).

Now that the patents for several of the original analog insulins have expired, biosimilar versions are being developed, which will become available over the next few years.

Fast-acting insulin can be the "magic bullet" when it comes to controlling blood sugars. Used properly, fast-acting insulin can eliminate dangerous post-meal spikes. Many people with Type 2 Diabetes will find that when they control post-meal spikes their fasting blood sugar will decrease, too. So after they add a fast-acting insulin to their regimen they need a lot less basal insulin.

But in order to use fast-acting insulin correctly, you have to match your dose to the amount of carbohydrate in your meal. Not only that, but because each person has a different level of sensitivity to insulin, you have to figure out, with the help of your doctor or a Certified Diabetes Educator, how many grams of carbohydrate one unit of insulin will cover. Match your insulin to the carbs in your food properly and you will see relatively flat, near normal post-meal blood sugars. But when dosing fast-acting insulin you have to always err on the side of caution, because if you use too much fast-acting insulin you can have very nasty hypos.

Dr. Bernstein makes the point in his book, *Dr. Bernstein's Diabetes Solution,* that the only way to use fast-acting insulin safely is to use it with a lowered carbohydrate intake. This is because the more carbohydrate you eat, the more likely you are to be wrong when you estimate how many grams of carbohydrate are on your plate. And the more wrong you are about how much carbohydrate you are eating, the more likely you are to inject the wrong dose of insulin.

Another problem with injected fast-acting insulin involves the speed with which it is absorbed from the injection site into the blood. The larger the dose, the slower it may be absorbed. Ideally you want the glucose from your food to hit the bloodstream at the same time as the insulin does. To make that happen, you must be aware of the absorption speed of the particular insulin you are injecting—they are all slightly different—and must know how fast the food you ate will digest.

This is why meal-time insulin is tricky. Let's say you want to eat a plate of spaghetti and sauce. You estimate that it contains 80 grams of carbohydrate. Your CDE told you that, for you, one unit of insulin should cover 5 grams of carbohydrate. So you inject 16 units of Novolog, which usually starts to work by 15 minutes after you eat. But because pasta digests very slowly, that insulin may arrive in the bloodstream long before the glucose from the pasta gets there. Now you have 16 units of insulin in your bloodstream but almost no glucose for it to work on, so you end up with a hypo.

Alternatively, you may inject enough of the slower human insulin, Novolin R, to match the 70 grams of glucose contained in a bagel, only to discover that the bagel digested so quickly that the glucose from it hit your bloodstream *before* all the insulin was absorbed from the injection site. This will cause you to experience a high blood sugar spike. Then, a few hours later when all the insulin has been absorbed from that injection site, you may experience low blood sugar. This can happen because like most Type 2s, you still produce a small second-phase insulin release that may kick in occasionally—and unpredictably—after you eat. If that second-phase insulin release mops up some of the glucose from the bagel before the delayed injected insulin gets to it, you'll end up with more insulin in your system than glucose, and then, once again, it's hypo time.

And this doesn't even get into the question of what happens if that plate of spaghetti you ate only contained 50 grams of carbohydrate instead of the 80 grams you dosed for.

This should make it clear why using fast-acting insulin to cover meals is tricky. It also makes it clear why smart insulin users keep their carbohydrate intake relatively low. A lower carbohydrate content requires a smaller insulin dose. And when you use a small dose of fast-acting insulin with a relatively low intake of carbohydrate, if you don't quite match the insulin to the food, the insulin you've injected is not as likely to cause a serious hypo or leave you with a serious blood sugar spike.

This also should make it clear that it takes time to learn to use fast-acting insulin. Doctors and diabetes educators can give you some useful rules of thumb, but you will have to carefully observe your body's reaction to different doses used at different meals, and test your blood sugar after each meal over a period of months to really get the hang of using fast-acting insulin.

Don't be surprised if you find you need more insulin to cover breakfast than you do the identical food eaten at dinner. Our insulin resistance often varies throughout the course of the day. But if you have the patience to learn how to use fast-acting insulin, you can get extremely good control. Many of us do and are very grateful for it.

More Concentrated Forms of Insulin for High Insulin Resistance

People who are extremely insulin resistant may need huge doses of any of the insulins we have discussed. I have heard from people who were using as many as 300 units a day of basal insulin and still not getting good control. Such people may benefit from using a special formulation of R insulin that is highly concentrated. This insulin is called U500 R insulin. It contains five times as much insulin in a single unit, by volume, as does the U100 insulin normally prescribed. A person who needs to inject 300 units a day of Lantus would only need to inject 60 units of U500 R insulin. And because the U500 R insulin is so concentrated, it absorbs faster and does a better job of lowering blood sugar. If you are having difficulty getting a regular basal insulin to work, even at very high doses, you may have to visit an expert endocrinologist practicing at a teaching hospital to get U500 R insulin, as local endocrinologists don't often prescribe it.

The newest patented basal insulins are also available in more concentrated forms. Tresiba can be dispensed in either a standard U100 form or in a U200 version that is twice as concentrated. Toujeo is a U300 version of Lantus, which is three times as concentrated, though the pens it is sold in don't take advantage of this feature and still require that a person needing a large dose do multiple injections.

Premixed Insulins

Doctors sometimes start patients on so-called premixed insulins. These usually have the phrase "70/30" in their names. Premixed insulins are a mixture of fast and slow acting insulins. The "30" in the name refers to the 30% of the insulin that is fast-acting. The other 70% is a longer-acting insulin, either NPH or a longer-acting insulin made by adding zinc and protamine to Novolog or Humalog to slow them down. The newest premixed insulin, Ryzodeg, combines Tresiba, the new patented basal insulin and Novolog. There is also a 50/50 insulin available, Humalog Mix 50/50.

In theory, these mixed insulins save you money and make it possible to use fewer shots. But because you can't match the fast-acting component of the insulin to the carbohydrate content of your meals without also modifying the dose of the longer acting basal component, it's hard to get good blood sugar control using a premixed insulin. This is especially true if the long-acting component of the insulin is NPH or a protamine version of a fast-acting insulin, since these protamine insulins are notorious for causing hypos. Ryzodeg 70/30 may be less likely to cause hypos, because the long-acting component, Tresiba has a much smoother activity curve. But it will still be impossible to match the fast-acting component in Ryzodeg to the carbohydrate content of your meals. If your doctor prescribes this kind of insulin, give it a try, but if you have trouble making it work, ask your doctor to prescribe separate basal and fast-acting insulins so you can adjust the doses of the two kinds of insulin separately and get them right.

Basal Insulins Mixed with GLP-1 Agonists

Several products that were approved in Europe in 2014 and are awaiting approval in the United States combine basal insulin with a GLP-1 receptor agonist. These include Xultophy, which is a mixture of Tresiba and Victoza, and Lixilan, which is a mixture of Lantus and Lyxumia. Even for those who are not deterred by the problems associated with the GLP-1 receptor agonists that we discussed in the previous chapter, these are a poor choice. Adding the GLP-1 receptor agonist to a basal insulin makes it harder to adjust the dose of the basal insulin to fit a person's very individual requirements. Raising the dose so that enough basal insulin is delivered to control the needs of a very insulin resistant person may result in also delivering a very high dose of the GLP-1 receptor agonist, which will raise the possibility of side effects that can include nausea and vomiting, and of course, increasing the possibility of stimulating abnormal growth of cells in the pancreas.

Inhaled Ultra Fast-Acting Insulin

A new, ultra fast-acting insulin, Afrezza (generic name, Technosphere insulin), was approved for sale in the United States in 2014. Unlike the other insulins we have been discussing, it comes in powder form and is inhaled rather than injected. Afrezza is made out of molecules of regular human insulin that have been coated with a chemical that dissolves when it reaches the lung tissue. This allows the insulin molecule to be quickly absorbed by the blood vessels concentrated there.

Afrezza is very fast. It starts to work fifteen minutes after it is inhaled and is completely gone two hours later. This means that unlike the injected fast-acting insulins, Afrezza comes much closer to mimicking *first-phase* insulin release rather than second-phase. Rumor has long had it that other ultra-fast insulins are under development, but for now, none appears close to approval. So Afrezza is unique in filling this role.

Unfortunately, few doctors seem aware of the value of having an insulin that replaces a missing first-phase insulin release and few insurers cover it at a tier that makes it affordable. That's because the trial data submitted to the FDA when Afrezza came up for approval did not demonstrate that Afrezza was better than injected fast-acting insulin at lowering A1c. It only showed that Afrezza was slightly more effective than *no* insulin in people with Type 2 Diabetes who had failed to achieve even mediocre control with oral drugs.

Only a few thousand people have tried Afrezza, and most of them have Type 1 Diabetes. So there is currently not enough user feedback for us to be able to determine how well it really works for people with Type 2 diabetes. Given that it replaces first-phase rather than second-phase insulin, it should be most helpful for people with mild to moderate Type 2 Diabetes who still can make some second-phase insulin. Unfortunately, most insurers will only cover it for people with Type 2 Diabetes who have already failed to achieve control when taking several oral drugs. They have had diabetes for so long that they have lost most of their second-phase insulin release.

Afrezza is packaged in disposable cartridges that you drop into a small inhaler that looks a lot like a whistle. The cartridges range in size from 4 to 12 units. Each box of Afrezza contains 90 cartridges. All but the 4 unit boxes contain a mix of large and small cartridges. This makes it difficult for people with Type 2 Diabetes who need large doses of insulin at every meal to use Afrezza, as it is not currently possible to get a box made up of only the 12 unit cartridges.

User reports suggest that Afrezza doses, though expressed in units, do not behave like the same number of units of injected insulin would. So it may take some experimentation to determine the proper dose to use. Afrezza is supposed to be inhaled at the beginning of a meal. Some users report that Afrezza finishes working so quickly that they may have to use a second dose an hour after eating to cover the rest of the glucose from the meal. Others find they do better if they inhale Afrezza a few minutes after they start eating.

Afrezza Side Effects

The most common side effect of Afrezza is coughing after inhalation. Because of this, the FDA mandates that you must take a pulmonary function test before your doctor can prescribe it for you. You will also need to get your lung function rechecked periodically after starting the drug, to ensure that it doesn't cause your lung function to decline. The manufacturer claims that any decline that might happen is reversible upon stopping use, but until the drug has a longer history, this assurance can't be relied on. Afrezza should also not be prescribed to smokers.

Afrezza may turn out to be a very useful tool for lowering blood sugar, but it is too new for us to know what the long-term side effects are. That will only become known after thousands of patients use it for years. So, as is the case with any new drug, it may be best to wait a few years and let others be the guinea pigs who determine its true value.

Treating Hypos

Everyone who is using insulin should learn how to treat hypos. A mild hypo may occur when you have taken slightly more insulin than you needed. Your doctor should tell you at what blood sugar level you should correct a mild hypo. For many of us, that level is below 80 mg/dl. There is no need to correct blood sugars in the 80s unless your blood sugar is dropping quickly and you know your insulin will not stop working for a while longer.

Serious hypos are those where your blood sugar drops below 50 mg/dl. They usually occur when you have injected a much larger dose of insulin than you intended or have mistakenly injected fast-acting insulin instead of your basal insulin. Accidentally injecting basal insulin into a vein can also cause severe hypos.

People taking beta blockers to control their blood pressure or protect their hearts after a heart attack are more likely to experience hypos, as these drugs turn off the protective mechanism your body normally uses to raise your blood sugar as you begin to hypo. If you are experiencing hypos and take one of these drugs, talk to your doctor about switching to a different kind of drug.

Always check your blood sugar before driving a car and be sure your blood sugar is at a safe level before you set out. Having a hypo while driving can kill you, your passengers, and innocent bystanders.

Glucose is the Best Treatment for Hypos

You should correct hypos with glucose, not food. There are two grams of glucose in five American "Smarties" candy discs or one hard "Sweetarts" candy wafer. It is listed as "dextrose" on the label. Check the nutritional information on the wrapper to be sure this is still true as candy companies sometimes change their formulas or product sizes. You can also buy glucose tablets at the drug store. However, the good thing about Smarties and Sweetarts is that in an emergency you can buy them at gas stations and convenience stores. If you use insulin, keep glucose tabs or a roll of these candies in your pocket, purse, and car at all times.

The amount of glucose that raises your blood sugar a given amount depends on your body weight. Use Table 5 on the next page to find the amount of glucose you will need to eat to raise your blood sugar 10 mg/dl.

To treat a severe hypo, take enough glucose to raise your blood sugar by 70 mg/dl immediately. A sugary soda or orange juice will work in an emergency when you have no glucose. So will hard candies but not chocolates.

Test your blood sugar in 15 minutes, and if your blood sugar is not over 90 mg/dl take more glucose. If your blood sugar continues dropping steeply get someone to drive you to an emergency room.

The best way to treat a mild hypo is to take a small dose of pure glucose just large enough to raise your blood sugar from its current level to 110 mg/dl. Wait fifteen minutes and measure your blood sugar again. It should be where you wanted it to be unless whatever caused your hypo is still having an effect. If it is still in the hypo range, take another dose of the size that should raise it to 110 mg/dl.

Your Weight (lbs)	Glucose Needed (g)
140	2
175	2.5
210	3
245	3.5
280	4
315	4.5

Table 5. Glucose Needed to Raise Blood Sugar 10 mg/dl

Why Not Just Eat Two Grams of High Carb Food?

It is best to use pure glucose because it is the only sugar that goes directly into your blood stream and does not require the time-consuming digestion that sucrose, lactose, fructose, or starch require. Glucose is already in the form that goes into the bloodstream.

If you try to raise your blood sugar with starchy or sugary food or with proteins or fats that will slow its digestion.

If you have been restricting your carbs very tightly, you may look upon a mild hypo as an opportunity to eat a high carbohydrate treat, such as a piece of cake. This is a bad habit to get into. Treat hypos with speedy glucose. If you want a piece of cake, schedule an off-plan indulgence. Eating sugary food to counter frequent mild hypos can cause weight gain. There are only four calories in a gram of glucose. So even if you take 12 grams, you are only going to get 48 calories. But if you start eating starchy and sugary food to correct frequent hypos, you are likely to eat far more calories. Over time those calories will add up. This may be another reason why drugs that cause hypos, like insulin and sulfonylureas are associated with weight gain.

Chapter Eleven
Supplements and Healing Foods

Can Special Foods and Supplements Control Diabetes?

Because cutting down on carbohydrates makes such a huge difference in your blood sugars, it's easy to believe there must be other foods and supplements that would have an equally powerful effect and might even be powerful enough to let you work that fudge sundae back into your food plan.

But such foods and supplements don't exist. What does exist is a huge industry looking to make money off you and other people with chronic diseases, an industry that profits mightily from selling you worthless remedies at highly inflated prices. Many of them are advertised using Google and Facebook ads. Paid shills also tout their benefits on online discussion forums. These remedies line the shelves of so-called "Health Food" stores, and puff-pieces about them fill many pages of magazines devoted to health and fitness.

If you're newly diagnosed, it's almost certain that you are going to shell out for some of them. They promise so much, and you're only human! But before you head down to the health food store and drain your bank account, consider the following.

Why You Need to Be Suspicious of Dietary Research Boosting Specific Foods and Supplements

Though the media often report that one or another food or supplement prevents or cures diabetes, these reports are almost always based on company-issued press releases. These tout the findings of studies the makers of these products commission from research mills—companies that guarantee a positive result to anyone willing to pay for it. Often the study has been published in a vanity journal, one that will publishes any study, no matter how awful, in return for a hefty fee. The press rarely reports on the work of the independent academic researchers who call these claims into question or disprove them.

For example, while you've undoubtedly read many articles suggesting that eating soy products can help women with menopausal symptoms, you probably missed the research that showed that those same soy products can be toxic to the thyroid glands of those same menopausal women or that eating soy products may make you more susceptible to developing food allergies. Nor are you likely to have read about the research done by scientists *not* funded by the soy producers that casts doubt on whether soy really is effective for countering menopausal symptoms. (It isn't.)

There are virtually no investigative journalists working in the medical press. Newspapers and TV networks simply print the press releases companies mail them without making any attempt to check their validity. When a doctor is quoted in these press releases-turned-into-news items, it is almost always a doctor on the payroll of the company who sent out the press release.

The Supplement Business Is Rife with Fraud

Even if a supplement really lives up to its health claims, there is no guarantee that the product you paid for is in the capsule that you bought. In fact, it's likely that it isn't. That's because the supplement business in the United States is completely unregulated.

Lab analyses run by watchdog groups often find that bottles of supplements contain a lot less of the supplement than what is listed on the label. Even worse, they often contain other substances *not* listed on the label, some of which may be harmful. To cite only one example, in 2011, a large "well respected" Utah supplement company marketed a product, Zotrex, supposedly containing an natural herb, *ophioglossum polyphyllous*, which it claimed could enhance sexual potency. What the pills actually contained was sulfoaildenafil, a drug analog of Viagra that has never been tested in humans.

In another case, when a supposedly "herbal" diabetes supplement was taken to the lab, it turned out to contain a cheap first generation sulfonylurea drug—one that can cause dangerous hypos and acts on the heart in a way that promotes heart attack.

In 2015, the New York State Attorney General's Office conducted tests using sophisticated DNA technology to see what was really in herbal capsules. They found that 79% of store brand herbal supplements sold in Walmart, Target, Walgreens, and GNC either didn't contain the stated ingredient(s), or were contaminated by other filler materials such as rice and wheat, to which some people might be allergic. Similar studies in the past have found the same degree of contamination in products sold by many other herbal supplement vendors. Some contained grass clippings instead of the costly herb on the label. Others contained dangerous substances.

A 1994 law stipulated that supplement makers were supposed to submit safety data to the FDA for any new ingredient they introduced that wasn't on sale prior to 1994. But the *New England Journal of Medicine* reported in 2012 that since 1994,

> ... the number of available dietary supplements has skyrocketed from an estimated 4000 to more than 55,000 ... but the FDA has received adequate notification for only 170 new supplement ingredients since 1994 — undoubtedly a small fraction of the ingredients for which safety data should have been submitted.

A major problem with herbal supplements is that while they may be "natural" that doesn't mean they don't contain substances that might be bad for you. For example, there are several Chinese herbs that are effective in lowering blood sugar. They do this because they contain naturally occurring sulfonylurea molecules. So they also stimulate receptors on your heart in the same way that first generation sulfonylurea drugs did — a way that increases your likelihood of having a heart attack.

Red rice yeast lowers cholesterol because it contains a naturally-occurring statin molecule. So it will also cause all the nasty side effects of a prescription statin. The only difference between taking these "natural" supplements and a prescription drug is that when you take the supplement version you don't know what substance you are actually ingesting. The lack of regulation also means that even if the pill does contain the supplement listed on the label, the dose of the effective component in the supplement may vary greatly from pill to pill, even in a single bottle.

Questionable Supplements

With these warnings in mind, lets look at some of the foods and supplements that are touted as helping you control your blood sugar. We will start with the most popular — and least effective.

Cinnamon

Cinnamon is a perennial favorite of those seeking "natural" diabetes cures. The idea that cinnamon might have some effect on blood sugar was first demonstrated in 1990 at a lab run by Dr. Richard A. Anderson of the Human Nutrition Research Center of the FDA in Beltsville Maryland. It was testing foods for an insulin-enhancing effect as part of a series of studies. Cinnamon was only one of several foods they described as having an insulin-enhancing effect. Others included peanut butter and tuna fish. The article reporting these results was published in an obscure journal and attracted no media attention.

Dr. Anderson's very small studies that found a favorable effect from cinnamon only measured *fasting blood sugar* and were conducted in people without diabetes. When other researchers examined the effect of cinnamon on people with diabetes the title of their study says it all: "Cinnamon supplementation does not improve glycemic control in postmenopausal Type 2 Diabetes patients." That study included glucose tolerance test results in its assessment of the efficacy of cinnamon.

Another study found that cinnamon doesn't even improve fasting blood sugars. This study, performed by researchers at the University of Oklahoma randomly assigned people with Type 2 Diabetes to take either cinnamon capsules or a placebo every day for three months. The cinnamon group took two capsules a day, each of which contained 500 milligrams of the spice. The placebo group took capsules containing wheat flour. The results of this study showed that there were no differences in the groups' average levels of blood sugar, insulin, or cholesterol.

Cinnamon does have the advantage that you can test it at home safely and cheaply. Keep your dose to one teaspoon a day or less, and if you have high blood pressure be sure to monitor it. Contrary to Dr. Anderson's claims that cinnamon lowers blood pressure, some people who have tested it have reported seeing their blood pressure go up after taking cinnamon. Do not use cinnamon if you have any issues related to bleeding, as cinnamon contains a substance related to coumarin, a blood thinner.

And don't bother with those $30 bottles of cinnamon extract sold by supplement companies. They may claim that their products contain exotic forms of cinnamon that differ from what you can buy at the grocery store. But Dr. Anderson has stated in interviews that cassia — the stuff you buy at the grocery store labeled "cinnamon" — is what he and his students used in the original research that found benefits from taking cinnamon.

Chromium

There was a flurry of excitement about chromium in the 1990s, after the same Dr. Anderson who got such impressive results with cinnamon reported that chromium supplementation could significantly improve glucose tolerance. Studies conducted by Dr. Anderson and other researchers around the world seemed to show that adding chromium to the diets of people with diabetes in India and China lowered their blood sugar significantly. However, other studies with European and American populations did not show chromium having any such effect.

In his review of the chromium studies published in the *Journal of the American College of Nutrition* in 1998, Anderson argued that to be effective chromium should be given in the form of chromium picolinate rather than less active chromium chloride and that the minimum dose must be at least 400 micrograms and possibly as much as 1,000. This dose, he said could reduce insulin resistance in people with impaired glucose tolerance and lower the blood sugar of people with Type 2 Diabetes. Anderson explained that the mechanism behind this improvement was that chromium supplementation increases the number of insulin receptors in cells.

However, despite Anderson's enthusiasm for chromium — his name was on many of the relevant research papers — none of these studies were particularly impressive. All were small. None of them involved more than 85 people and few involved more than 30.

The media — probably responding to press releases from supplement manufacturers — picked up on this and other research in 1998 and publicized it in a way that suggested that chromium supplementation not only would reduce insulin resistance but that it would also improve the speed with which dieters lost weight. Sales of chromium picolinate skyrocketed.

But few dieters found the supplement to be all that effective, and a subsequent review of the research by NIH statisticians, M.D. Althuis and N.E. Jordan concluded that chromium supplementation had no effect on glucose or insulin levels in non-diabetic people and that the evidence for an effect on people with diabetes was inconclusive.

Some researchers speculated that the results seen in the Chinese and Indian studies might have been due to these particular populations subsisting on mediocre diets that were deficient in chromium. The diet eaten by most people in the First World supplies more than enough chromium.

If you want to test chromium you can buy inexpensive chromium picolinate at the drug store. Try one package and if you don't see a significant change, you'll know it isn't worth investing in.

Even better, the safest approach to chromium supplementation — as is the case with most mineral supplementation — is to get chromium from the foods you eat. Foods rich in chromium that won't raise your blood sugar include seafood, green beans, broccoli, nuts, and peanut butter, all of which contain other helpful micronutrients. Eating foods that contain vitamin C, like berries or green pepper, may increase the absorption of dietary chromium.

If a supplement company claims you can't get the health benefits of some nutrient by eating several servings a day of foods that contain it, be skeptical. Over and over again research comes up with the finding that nutrients originally identified as having health benefits when they were taken in the form of food are worthless when taken in pills.

For example, people eating a lot of vegetables containing beta carotene appeared to suffer less lung cancer than those who did not. But when the beta carotene was administered in the form of vitamin pills no such effect was observed. There are many micronutrients in real foods, which are not included in pills, and it's possible they work together synergistically.

Antioxidant Vitamins

Many small scale studies appeared to show that the antioxidant vitamins C and E might help prevent heart disease. However, a large scale study conducted in England, where half of 20,536 people considered at high risk for heart disease took vitamin C, E, and beta-carotene supplements and half didn't, cast a great deal of doubt on this. Despite the fact that those in the supplemented group had measurably higher blood levels of the supplemented vitamins, the researchers found no difference at all in their rates of heart attack, other signs of cardiovascular disease, cancer or, indeed, hospitalization for any other cause.

A separate study published in 2007 found that antioxidant supplements actually seemed to *raise* the risk of death in those who took them. Additional research published in 2015 cast more light on the mechanism by which antioxidants might increase mortality. They found that cancer cells usually experience a very high level of oxidative stress, which kills them, but when mice were transplanted with human melanoma cells, giving them antioxidants lowered that stress, keeping the cancerous cells alive and growing.

Some still believe that supplementing with these vitamins might be of some use to people with diabetes. Studies have certainly shown that the beta cell is uniquely vulnerable to oxidative stress because it is poor at producing antioxidant substances. So it has seemed reasonable to think that raising the bloodstream concentrations of these antioxidants might help counter this. But careful analysis of data from the EPIC Norfolk study, which had concluded that higher blood levels of Vitamin C correlated with lower A1cs, found that the only reason for this correlation was that a high blood level of Vitamin C was a marker for having the higher income that allowed for a healthier way of eating. The study title says it all: "Occupational social class, educational level and area deprivation independently predict plasma ascorbic acid concentration." In short, the better off and the better educated you are, the more likely you are to eat a diet filled with the fresh fruits and vegetables that will raise the level of vitamin C in your blood, rather than a cheaper diet filled with starchy, sugary junk food that will raise your blood sugar.

Vitamin E Appears Effective in the Presence of a Certain Gene

One reason for the confusing results described above in large-scale studies of antioxidants became clear in 2007. A team in Israel discovered that people with one particular gene, the haptoglobin (Hp) 2-2 gene, who took 400 IU of Vitamin E, had 40% less heart attacks over an 18 month period than those who did not have that particular gene. So this supplement may have benefits for a subset of people.

All this should make it clear that if you feel you must take these vitamins in supplemental form, use low doses. Dr. Bernstein warns against taking doses of vitamin C greater than 500 mg a day, explaining that very high levels of vitamin C can raise blood sugar and impair nerve function. He writes that vitamin E in doses between 400 to 1,200 IU per day may lower insulin resistance, but suggests you use gamma tocopherol or mixed tocopherols, not the commonly found version of Vitamin E, alpha tocopherol, which he says can inhibit the absorption of gamma tocopherol from food.

Get Your Antioxidants from Food

Because of the fraud so common in the supplement business and because your body evolved over millions of years during which nutrients did not arrive in the form of pills, you are much more likely to get whatever health benefits there are in any nutrient if you get that nutrient from eating the foods where it naturally occurs in the doses your body evolved to handle. To get antioxidants from food, consume nuts and sunflower seeds, which are an excellent source of vitamin E. You can get adequate amounts of vitamin C from green vegetables, small servings of tomato, and low carbohydrate fruits like blueberries, raspberries, and strawberries.

Vitamin D

Vitamin D, despite its name, is a hormone not a vitamin. It plays a major role in the regulation of blood calcium levels and bone strength. Hope that Vitamin D might be a treatment for diabetes rose after a study published in 2007 found that in a population of roughly 4,000 Finnish men and women, individuals with higher blood levels of Vitamin D had a 40 percent lower risk of developing Type 2 Diabetes than did those with lower levels of this vitamin. The next year another study documented that low levels of Vitamin D also correlated with a higher risk of heart disease. But subsequent studies that attempted to lower people's blood sugar by giving them Vitamin D failed to produce any positive results, and a study of 446 European subjects diagnosed with metabolic syndrome found no relationship between their blood concentrations of Vitamin D and their insulin secretion or sensitivity.

This suggests that something about the conditions that lead to the development of diabetes lowers Vitamin D levels, rather than that a deficiency of Vitamin D causes diabetes.

The sole research evidence that Vitamin D may be useful to people with diabetes comes from a study published in 2008 that found that patients with chronic kidney disease given Calcitriol (a form of Vitamin D) had a 26% lower mortality and a 20% lower rate of going onto dialysis over a period of almost two years. But to date there is no evidence that supplementing with Vitamin D improves or prevents any of the many other conditions where sufferers are found to have low levels of the hormone.

Not only does supplemental Vitamin D not improve the health of people with diabetes, but as large numbers of people began supplementing with Vitamin D doctors began to see a revival of what used to be a rare condition, Milk Alkali syndrome, which can be fatal. This is a condition where blood calcium levels rise extremely high. It is caused by exposure to too much Vitamin D. But too much Vitamin D can be a problem even for people who don't develop this rare condition. It turns out that even blood levels of Vitamin D well within the range flagged as normal on blood tests can result in high blood calcium levels. This is a problem since blood calcium levels at the high end of the range labs label "normal" turn out to correlate with higher blood pressure and an elevated risk of coronary artery disease.

This makes it essential that if you decide to supplement with this hormone you get your blood levels of Vitamin D and calcium checked before you begin supplementation and periodically after that. My endocrinologist informed me that doctors are coming to think that blood levels of Vitamin D that reach the high 50 ng/ml range, are not healthy. Levels of 89 ng/ml correlate with a significantly raised risk of heart disease.

Also be aware that Vitamin D levels are reported using two kinds of units. The ng/mL unit used in most United States labs gives a reading that must be multiplied by 2.6 to give the nmol/L value you see reported in many, but not all, research studies. Raising levels reported in mg/dl to the levels cited in research studies that use the nmol/L units will result in your having abnormally high, and possibly dangerous blood levels of Vitamin D.

Some proponents of supplementation—some of whom earn big bucks selling their own brands of supplements—believe that taking Vitamin K2 can prevent the accumulation of calcium in the arteries caused by taking too much Vitamin D or even reverse it. But why attempt to prevent the damage caused by one questionable, unregulated supplement by taking another? It makes more sense to monitor your Vitamin D levels and only supplement when they are low. If you do supplement, stick with the 1,000 IU dose rather than megadoses.

Magnesium

An analysis of data from the Nurses Health Study suggested that increased intake of dietary magnesium corresponded with a reduced risk of diabetes. This result was echoed by a similar finding analyzing data from another study, the Iowa Women's Health Study. Adequate blood levels of magnesium have also been found to counter high blood pressure.

However, again it is not clear whether high blood magnesium levels truly prevent blood sugar deterioration or are simply a marker that a person does not have the underlying conditions that cause abnormal blood sugars.

A new concern about supplementing minerals, including magnesium, is the finding published in 2008 that calcium supplementation at the high levels recommended at the time appeared to increase the incidence of heart attacks in older women. This may be because excess calcium gets deposited as hard plaque in the arteries.

Since blood magnesium levels affect calcium levels, it may be a mistake to supplement either of these minerals with pills. Get your magnesium from the nuts and leafy green vegetables you should be eating for all the other good things they contain. Plentiful amounts of magnesium are also found in premium chocolates with high cocoa content.

Dangerous Trace Minerals

Selenium is a trace mineral that had been found in some small experiments to appear to lower blood sugar. However, a study published in 2007 attempted to see whether long-term supplementation with selenium would prevent Type 2 Diabetes. It concluded that it appeared to do just the opposite. The group taking the selenium supplements developed more diabetes. Not only that, but the more selenium in their blood plasma, the more likely people were to develop diabetes. Strike selenium off your list of supplements for diabetes, unless you want to *get* diabetes.

Another trace mineral, which you will see touted for blood sugar control by the sleazy doctors who earn their livings not from treating patients but from selling overpriced supplements on the web, is vanadyl sulfate, a vanadium compound. There is no question that vanadyl sulfate simulates the behavior of insulin and lowers blood sugar. The problem is with how it does it.

Dr. Sreedhara at Ohio State has done extensive work testing this supplement on rodents and has found that it damages DNA, blocks protein synthesis, and oxidizes lipids, which contributes to the development of cardiovascular disease. In addition, contrary to what you may read on supplement-selling web sites, these disturbing effects are seen at normal physiologic levels similar to those that would be expected to occur after taking the supplements available at health food stores. Even worse, other research has found that vanadyl sulfate kills beta cells.

If you aren't making enough insulin, rather than experiment with minerals whose long-term side effects have never been tested in humans, are poorly understood, and may be very harmful, ask your doctor to let you supplement with real insulin or take repaglinide, the one reasonably safe, short-acting, insulin-stimulating drug whose possible side effects are well-understood.

Herbs

You'll often see the herbs gymnema sylvestre, berberine, and the Indian spice, fenugreek touted as being able to lower blood sugar. You can try sprinkling fenugreek on your food to see if it helps you. It is sold as a spice and it can be found in fresh form at Indian grocery stores. The fresh leaves are preferable, as they are eaten as a normal part of diets in some parts of the world, and there is anecdotal evidence that eating the leaves may lower blood sugar.

But here, as in the case of most herbs, there is always the possibility that these herbs lower blood sugar in ways that are not good for you, for example, by over-stimulating the beta cells. As noted diabetes author Gretchen Becker has pointed out, many "natural" cures popular in India work because they damage the liver. When the liver is damaged it no longer dumps glucose into your bloodstream, so your blood sugar drops. Unfortunately, as the damage continues, your liver no longer removes toxins from your blood and, barring a liver transplant, you die. Until the mechanisms that allow these herbs to lower blood sugar are better understood, it's probably wise to avoid them.

Berberine is a Chinese herb that is heavily promoted on the web by the sleazy doctors with no training in endocrinology who make their living by selling overpriced, personally-branded supplements to people looking for a fast and easy miracle cure. They cite many studies to prove its effectiveness. However, there is only one study of berberine that was published in a reputable journal. That study showed that berberine did lower blood sugar effectively, but the study only lasted three months, which is nowhere near long enough to prove the herb's safety. And of course, since berberine is an imported herb often sourced from China where herbs are frequently adulterated with pesticides, herbicides, and hidden cheap pharmaceutical drugs no longer sold in the United States, you have no idea what you are really getting when you buy a berberine supplement.

Pure berberine should also be treated with caution as it affects the liver in a way that can block the elimination of many other drugs, including some statins, blood pressure medications, sleeping pills, and antibiotics. So taking berberine with these other medications can be dangerous. Berberine is also very dangerous for pregnant women and newborns as it prevents the liver from breaking down bilirubin, leading to a condition that can be toxic to fetuses and breastfeeding babies.

Possibly Helpful Supplements

The supplements we are about to discuss next are those where either peer-reviewed research or anecdotal reports from trusted sources support the idea that they may help people with diabetes.

Benfotiamine

Benfotiamine is a lipid soluble form of thiamine or vitamin B1. There is some reputable research suggesting that it might be helpful for people with diabetes. In particular it appears to help neuropathic pain and may reduce the incidence of microvascular complications. Other research suggests that thiamine can block the processes that lead to the microvascular complications: neuropathy, retinopathy, and kidney disease. Though peer-reviewed research is far from unanimous in drawing these conclusions.

Recommended Dose:

The dose used in the experiments with humans that found benefits in benfotiamine varies. In one such study the dose was "two 50 mg benfotiamine tablets four times daily" (400 mg/day). In another it was "a combination of benfotiamine (100 mg) and pyridoxine hydrochloride [B6] (100 mg)" once a day.

Be Cautious Supplementing Other B Vitamins

It turns out that megadoses of Folic Acid, B6 and B-12 worsen the progress of diabetic kidney disease and raise the risk that people who have diabetic kidney disease will experience strokes.

So if you supplement with these B vitamins, don't use doses higher than the recommended daily requirements—which are quite low—no more than 2 mg for B6, 3 mcg for B-12, and 600 mcg for folic acid. Where possible, get your B vitamins from foods that contain it, like nuts, meats, spinach, and other green vegetables.

Alpha Lipoic Acid

This expensive supplement has been used in intravenous form to treat neuropathy in Germany. It is an insulin mimic—i.e. it appears to stimulate some of the same receptors insulin does. It is also an antioxidant.

In a German study, doctors from Buhl and City Hospital in Baden-Baden administered different dosages of oral ALA and placebo to 74 patients for four weeks. They then tested their insulin levels and found that the ability to take up glucose improved by an average of 27% in the people taking the ALA compared to the placebo group. All the dosages they tested appeared equally effective. The lowest dose used was 600 mg taken once a day. However, this is still a very small study, and a published review of other studies found less conclusive results for ALA taken orally rather than intravenously.

Dr. Bernstein writes that he has his patients take ALA in combination with Evening Primrose Oil to potentiate the action of insulin, whether it is the insulin produced by their own bodies or injected.

When I have scanned the web for discussions about this supplement I have not turned up much encouraging news about its effect on enhancing insulin sensitivity. Many people report that the combination of ALA and EPO caused them intolerable gastric distress. EPO was reported to cause mood swings by others. And almost no one reports seeing significant changes in blood sugar after taking this expensive supplement pair. However, some people with Type 2 Diabetes do report that ALA helps them with neuropathic pain and that it doesn't seem to matter whether they use the time release or regular form. There is an isomer of ALA, R-ALA, which is supposed to be more bio-available. Dr. Bernstein recommends using this form, which is marketed in the United States under the brand name, "Insulow."

One Caution About ALA

An editorial in the Japanese Journal 'Internal Medicine'" warns that in people with a specific genetic makeup that makes them extremely likely to develop autoimmune (Type 1) diabetes, ALA may provoke an antibody attack. The explanation for why this happens is that "α-lipoic acid (ALA) is reduced in the body to a sulfhydryl compound" and that sulfur rich compounds stimulate the immune attack. This does not appear to be a concern for people who do not have a strong family history of autoimmune diabetes.

Recommended Dose:

The Baden-Baden study cited above used 600 mg orally once a day. *Dr. Bernstein's Diabetes Solution* recommends two 100 mg tablets every 8 hours to be taken along with one 500 mg capsule of Evening Primrose oil.

Coenzyme Q10

Coenzyme Q10 is necessary for the proper function of mitochondria and it has been shown to be helpful in treating a rare form of genetic diabetes caused by mitochondrial dysfunction. Statins lower Coenzyme Q, so people who take statins are told to take this supplement.

Right after the most profitable of the statin drugs, Lipitor, lost patent protection, the medical community learned that taking statins raises the risk of developing diabetes by 27%. This may be because of the way that statins limit mitochondrial function. Since Coenzyme Q10 appears to be able to reverse this effect, it might undo any increase in blood sugar caused by statins.

Cortisone drugs, which can dramatically raise blood sugar, also appear to decrease mitochondrial efficiency. It is possible that Coenzyme Q10 may help reverse high blood sugars caused by cortisone drugs.

One study conducted in 1999 found a dose of 120 mg a day dramatically dropped fasting blood sugar. However, another study, conducted with people diagnosed with Type 2 Diabetes did not duplicate these results. After treatment with CoQ10, their average fasting blood sugar dropped only slightly and their average A1c actually deteriorated slightly. This study used a higher dose, 200 mg a day.

Recommended Dose

There is no harm in testing a low dose of CoQ10, though because it is an antioxidant, use it sparingly. Start with 50 mg/day of a gel or oil soluble version. If it is going to have any effect on your blood sugar levels, you should see them improve within a week or two. If you don't, there's no reason to take it.

Are "Superfoods" Really Super?

After your diabetes diagnosis, you'll be much more likely to notice the never-ending stream of reports in the media about how this or that "superfood" has healing properties. Can you really use dark chocolate to control your blood pressure and drink more coffee to keep your blood sugar in line?

Alas, the answer in every case is "No, not if you actually want to make significant improvements."

The research on which manufacturers base their claims is often seriously flawed and intentionally misleading, to the point where eating the foods they promote as being good for diabetes may actually worsen your condition.

A Perfect Example of a Perfectly Flawed Study: "Soy Yogurt Could Help Control Diabetes"

This news item, which was distributed by the AP in November of 2006, is a good example of how industry uses poorly conducted research to support specious health claims for questionable products. It was titled, "Soy Yogurt Could Help Control Diabetes" and its conclusion was that blueberry soy yogurt "controls diabetes" because it contains more of a specific phytochemical that inhibits the enzymes that break down sugar than do the other fruit yogurts it was compared to.

What's striking here is that the researchers drew their conclusion that their yogurt "controlled diabetes" by measuring the amount of this phytochemical in the yogurts. They did not observe the effect of the sugary fruit-filled yogurt on anyone's blood sugar. Since both regular and soy fruit yogurt are full of sugar—usually 23 grams per serving, any fruit-filled yogurt will raise blood sugar far beyond the ability of any phytochemical to lower it.

The researchers who performed this study also claimed that their soy blueberry yogurt lowered ACE, a hormone involved in the regulation of blood pressure, more than did other sugary yogurts. Perhaps it also lowered ACE levels a few micrograms more than did Milky Ways and chocolate cake. This does *not* make it a drug in food form.

The medical press publishes these kinds of studies without subjecting them to any kind of critical analysis. Company press releases are printed word for word as if they were a news story. By the time the story reaches the TV audience it has been stripped of any facts you could use to assess its validity.

The Glycemic Index Fails to Produce Health Outcomes

So-called "low glycemic" foods are another group of foods that you will often see promoted as health food. Unfortunately, they aren't.

The glycemic index was established by testing foods in people with completely normal blood sugars. It purportedly found that some high carbohydrate foods raised blood sugar less than others, though attempts to duplicate the findings of the original research failed. Different groups of people given the same foods used to define the original glycemic index produced different glycemic index values for those same foods.

The reason these supposedly low glycemic foods might not raise blood sugar could be that people with normal blood sugar will get a strong second-phase insulin response that will quickly dispose of any slow digesting carbohydrates. So starchy foods that digest slowly would not raise their blood sugar. But this would have little relevance for people with diabetes whose second-phase insulin production is inadequate.

But the idea that low glycemic foods were healthy for anyone took a blow when a study published in the highly respected *Journal of the American Medical Association* in 2014 found that a low glycemic diet didn't even improve the health of *normal* people. It concluded,

> In this 5-week controlled feeding study, diets with low glycemic index of dietary carbohydrate, compared with high glycemic index of dietary carbohydrate, did not result in improvements in insulin sensitivity, lipid levels, or systolic blood pressure. ... using glycemic index to select specific foods may not improve cardiovascular risk factors or insulin resistance.

Carbs are carbs. Whether they digest slowly or quickly, they still require the same amount of insulin to mop up the glucose they release into the blood. And every bit of excess glucose that isn't burned immediately is converted into fats that circulate in the liver and blood stream raising lipids and turning into body fat. Some people can tolerate high carb diets filled with slow-digesting foods, but there is no advantage to eating them.

"Healthy" Whole Grains

The same junk food manufacturers who promoted the manipulative, poor quality "science" that came up with the glycemic index have also sold the medical establishment on the dubious claim that there exist so called "healthy whole grains" and that people with diabetes should be eating a lot of them.

The grain industry has sponsored many studies purporting to prove that whole grains have enormous health benefits for people with diabetes. In all these studies the researchers compare a whole grain food with some highly processed junk food. So yes, a study may prove that a slice of whole grain toast is slightly easier on your blood sugar than a heaping bowl of Sugar Frosted Flakes. But if you were to compare a breakfast made up of whole grain toast and oatmeal to one containing a cheese omelet, the real effect of those "healthy" whole gains on your health would quickly become apparent.

Anyone with a blood sugar meter can quickly establish whether or not any supposedly healing food is healthy. If any supposedly healthy "superfood" raises your blood sugar over your blood sugar target, it isn't healthy.

Chapter Twelve
Exercise

Every book, every article, and every doctor will tell you that you should control your diabetes with "diet and exercise," and it is true that for many people exercise is a valuable tool for controlling blood sugar.

Exercise may increase the insulin sensitivity of your muscles both while you exercise and for a few hours afterwards. However, it is important to understand that it increases insulin sensitivity only by counteracting the secondary insulin resistance that is caused by having high blood sugars. Exercise cannot change innate insulin resistance caused by genetic flaws, be they inherited or caused by toxic exposures.

Exercise also builds more muscle. Having more muscle will help you burn off slightly more glucose while resting and it may also slightly increase your insulin sensitivity overall, again by lowering abnormally high blood sugars.

When I have polled people with diabetes online about how effective they have found exercise, the responses have been quite revealing, as they have shown that there is a sharp divide between those who see a dramatic difference in their blood sugar when they exercise regularly and those who don't. Some people with diabetes have found that exercise makes no difference in their blood sugar control at all, while others find that exercise after meals can lower their post-meal blood sugars to normal levels, even when they eat high carbohydrate meals.

These reported differences in people with diabetes's response to exercise may have something to do with the finding we discussed in Chapter Two that some people with diabetes have mitochondria that do not burn glucose properly. Since the benefits of exercise are based on raising the rate at which the mitochondria in the muscles burn glucose and fat, people with diabetes who have that kind of genetic flaw may not experience those benefits. People with diabetes who have normal mitochondria, however, are more likely to respond.

Your blood sugar meter will be able to tell you how effective exercise is for you. Try eating the same meal with and without post-meal exercise, and see how much of a difference exercising makes in your own post-meal blood sugars. If a brisk walk after dinner allows you to eat dessert and still keep your blood sugar at your target level, you may be one of the lucky people who doesn't have to be quite as disciplined about what they eat—as long as you stay disciplined about taking that post-meal walk.

Most people think that "exercise" means going to the gym, and indeed, for many people, the weight training and endurance aerobics you can do with the help of the machines you find at a gym may be helpful. But if you have had high blood sugars for a while and have long been sedentary, an aggressive program of gym exercise may leave you with serious injuries that make future exercise impossible.

Gym exercises can also raise your heart rate dramatically, which can pose a problem if you don't start out very gradually and improve your cardiovascular fitness in small steps. Be sure to get your doctor's approval before you start a new exercise regimen.

When you start a brand new exercise regimen use the readouts on aerobic exercise machines or a personal fitness monitor to keep an eye on your heart rate and make sure that it doesn't rise higher than 75% of the maximum heart rate that is safe for a person of your age. The American Heart Association states that a healthy person's maximum heart rate should be 220 minus their age. This is conservative but it is better to err on the side of caution if you have long been sedentary. If you have been diagnosed with heart disease you must ask your doctor what heart rate is safe for you.

If you haven't been exercising at all, when you start out doing aerobic exercise, keep your heart rate between 50-70% of your maximum heart rate, slowing down any time your heart rate exceeds that target. Then work your heart rate up gradually over a period of weeks.

The Best Exercise is Exercise that Avoids Injury

As we mentioned in Chapter Four, people with diabetes or prediabetes who have experienced years of undiagnosed high blood sugars are very prone to develop tendon and back problems because high blood sugars appear to cause tendons to become brittle or even turn into bone. There is also evidence that years of exposure to even slightly elevated blood sugars can cause abnormal thickening of tendons and weaken the material making up spinal discs, making them more likely to rupture.

Therefore, if you are an older person with diabetes who may have had undiagnosed high blood sugars for many years, you are more likely than your peers to have fragile tendons throughout your body or discs in your back that are just waiting for an excuse to rupture. So when you take up a new exercise program you must be very careful to avoid the kinds of exercise that puts abnormal stress on your tendons, joints, and spine.

Walking is better than running because it is much less likely to damage the tendons in your knees. If you lift weights, don't be overly zealous. Do enough to increase your fitness but avoid damaging those vulnerable shoulders, vertebral discs, and knees.

This can be difficult to achieve in the typical gym environment, where the emphasis is on selling classes and personal training services that encourage people to overdo it. It is not accidental that the number of people needing joint replacements by their 50s and even 40s has surged. It is the natural result of ordinary people being sold the idea that it is normal to run marathons and grow muscles like the Incredible Hulk.

So if you are new to the world of the gym, don't trust that the muscular young "instructors" at your gym know what they are talking about. Many are poorly paid and have received a very limited education in exercise physiology. Some may have no formal training at all save what they were taught by the owners of the gym. And even those who have degrees in exercise physiology may know nothing about the problems older people encounter when they exercise with fragile tendons or an iffy back. Since gyms make sure you sign papers that exempt them from any liability should you injure yourself using their equipment, there is no motivation for them to ensure that you only do the kinds of exercise that are safe for you.

That is why many people with diabetes, especially those who are older or who have not exercised in many years, are better off adopting daily walking programs rather than heading for the gym. Study after study shows that half an hour of brisk walking five times a week will give you all the physiological benefits of exercise without damaging your joints. Swimming is another very healthy, joint-friendly exercise.

10,000 Steps

Exercising for four or five 30 minute sessions every week, though beneficial for your overall health, is not likely to make much—or even any—difference in your blood sugar. What might be more effective is looking for ways to increase the energy you expend throughout the day. Some people with diabetes have found it very helpful to snap a pedometer on their belt and use it to count their steps. Their goal is to gradually increase the number of steps they take each day until they have gotten up to 10,000 steps.

Just tracking your activity level has been shown to motivate people to increase it. Walking a couple flights of stairs rather than taking an elevator, parking at the far end of the parking lot, and taking a break every so often to walk to the other side of the building where you work may not seem like an "exercise program," but it is actually more likely to improve your health over the long term because it builds new and better habits.

Fitbits and other personal activity trackers that connect with your smartphone via apps are a more high tech way of tracking your activity level, and may be even more motivating if you share your data with friends. There is nothing like a bit of friendly competition to make you pursue your goals.

The only issue to be aware of if you use a fitness tracker is that these devices only give you an estimate of calories burned, and some kinds of activity can generate falsely high calorie counts.

Get off Your Butt—Literally

There is some evidence that sitting, in and of itself, is damaging to our health. So another approach to exercise is to change the way you work and relax so that you stand more than you sit. Standing desks allow you to work on a computer while standing up and have been adopted by some workplaces because of the belief that they have health benefits. A two day study conducted among office workers in the UK found that three hours a day of working while standing made a significant decrease in subjects' post-meal blood sugar excursions starting at 50 minutes after eating. Standing also burnt off an additional 50 calories an hour.

Other brief studies have come up with similar findings, though there are no longer-lasting studies that might tell us whether this improvement persists after workers have adapted to working standing up. Studies of other kinds of exercise have found that due to something called "training effect," people who engage in the same exercise for several months burn less calories at the same level of exertion. Still, standing more is well worth a try.

Because working while standing has becoming popular you will see several companies selling very expensive standing desks. However, there is no need to buy any expensive equipment to test out whether this approach might work for you. You can easily make your own, homemade "standing desk" by raising your PC monitor, keyboard, and mouse off your regular desk using a combination of small boxes or thick books. If you work on a laptop, try putting your laptop on a small raised shelf. Googling "homemade standing desk" will turn up quite a few innovative solutions that others have come up with. I have been working at a standing desk for almost a year now and am impressed at how much better my neck and back feel after a day of work.

If you don't work at a desk or are retired, you can still take steps to increase how much time you spend standing. Reconfigure the space where you pursue your hobbies so you stand rather than sit. Stand up while using your smartphone. If you watch a lot of TV, consider redesigning the room where you watch so that you can comfortably watch the screen in a standing position rather than sprawled in a recliner.

When You Can't Exercise

If, like many older people, you have orthopedic problems that make it extremely difficult to exercise, you may become depressed by the thought that your lack of mobility means you won't be able to achieve the benefits that exercise may make possible. You may also worry that you won't be able to control your weight because you have been brainwashed to believe that weight loss requires exercise, but that turns out not to be true.

Exercise has many benefits, but it is nowhere near as helpful in attaining weight loss as the people selling gym memberships would have you believe. In fact, some studies show that people who exercise tend to greatly overestimate how many calories they burn. This leads them to overeat and end up with *less* success with weight control.

A book that followed successful dieters who had lost a lot of weight and kept it off more than five years found that few of the successful women dieters they interviewed had done any exercise until they reached their weight goals, though many of them used exercise to help them maintain their weight loss over time.

Not only can you lose weight with out exercise, but it is also possible to reach your blood sugar goals without it. I have heard from many people with diabetes who have been able to maintain normal blood sugars for at least three years without exercise.

So if your mobility is limited, don't panic. Do what you can. Walk, roll, or wiggle what you can wiggle. And stick to your diet!

Exercise and Blood Sugar Level

Exercise should leave you feeling energized. If you feel drained for many hours after completing your exercise session, it's quite possible your exercise regimen is negatively affecting your blood sugar in ways that call for adjustment.

Exercise will sometimes raise blood sugars. At other times it can cause hypos. The highs can result when intense exercise leads to the release of stress hormones. Since stress hormones also make you more insulin resistant for hours after you experience them, exercising in a way that raises blood sugars is a bad idea for people with diabetes.

It is also possible, when you do aerobic exercise starting with your blood sugar at a normal level, that you may end up with the symptoms of low blood sugar. This is more likely to happen if you are eating a low carb diet or taking metformin, both of which limit the ability of the liver to dump glucose into your blood stream to raise blood sugars when they drop below a normal level. This potential for hypos is of particular concern when you are using insulin or a drug that makes the beta cells secrete insulin.

To avoid these problems, use your meter to learn the impact of exercise on your own blood sugar. Test before you start your exercise session. Then check your blood sugar after every fifteen minutes of exercising or if you find yourself "hitting the wall" while doing strenuous aerobic activities. Check again when you finish and two hours later. If you see your blood sugar going up rather than down, you'd do better to find a less stressful form of exercise or increase the duration of your exercise rather than its intensity. If you see your blood sugar drop, you now have a helpful technique for correcting spikes caused by unwise eating. However, though if you see your blood sugar drop below 70 mg/dl go easy! Provoking hypos can cause bursts of stress hormones that will make you temporarily more insulin resistant.

Avoid the temptation to correct mild hypos you experience while exercising with sugary sports drinks or juices. These contain so much sugar that they can push your blood sugar way up. If your blood sugar goes way down and then way up while you exercise, you will not only end up making yourself more insulin resistant, you'll end up ravenously hungry.

Just as was the case with the diabetes diet, the key to long-term success with exercise is avoiding extremes. a good diabetes exercise program is one you can stick with for decades, long past the point where your initial enthusiasm wanes. Its also just as true for exercise as it is for diet that you are most likely to succeed at exercise over the long-term if you treat yourself gently and don't force yourself to do things you hate.

Find activities you enjoy that improve fitness, and when they get boring replace them with new ones. A steady program that increases your fitness in a modest way year in and year out is much better for a person with diabetes than indulging in a few months of aggressive over-exercising, burning out, injuring yourself, and going back to being sedentary!

Chapter Thirteen
Is It Really Type 2?

If you've been diagnosed with Type 2 Diabetes but have been diagnosed with another autoimmune condition or if you are not overweight and lack other markers of insulin resistance such as an apple-shaped distribution of body fat or a strong response to metformin, it's possible that you don't really have Type 2 Diabetes. This is especially likely if after you cut way back on your carbohydrates you are still experiencing high post-meal blood sugars. If you have relatives with autoimmune diseases, or who are also of normal weight but have been diagnosed with either Type 2 or Type 1 Diabetes, it is even more likely.

That's because there are two other forms of diabetes that are often misdiagnosed as Type 2 Diabetes. Many family doctors have not been trained to recognize them and may not even know they exist.

LADA

Latent Autoimmune Diabetes of Adults (LADA) is a slow-developing form of autoimmune diabetes that usually occurs in people over 30 years old. It is often misdiagnosed as Type 2.

Evidence is emerging that LADA, though it is an autoimmune disease, is not quite the same as the Type 1 Diabetes that strikes in childhood. Instead, it may share features of both Type 1 and Type 2. This was made clear in a study published in 2008. It reported that though people diagnosed with LADA had versions of the HLA autoimmunity genes that were similar to those found in people with Type 1 Diabetes, many also had versions of the TCF7L2 gene that have been associated with Type 2 Diabetes.

But because LADA is an autoimmune form of diabetes where beta cells are killed by autoimmune attacks over time, it is likely to progress to a condition indistinguishable from full-fledged Type 1 Diabetes. So if there is a chance that you might have LADA it is important to get the tests that could diagnose it or rule it out, since once your beta cells are wiped out, you can experience the life-threatening condition caused by extremely high blood sugars called diabetic ketoacidosis (DKA).

The symptoms of DKA include excessive thirst, frequent urination, nausea and vomiting, abdominal pain, shortness of breath, fruity-scented breath, and confusion. You should suspect DKA when your blood sugar remains consistently higher than 300 mg/dl over a period of several hours. If that happens, contact your doctor immediately or go to the emergency room. DKA can be fatal. If you experience DKA and are not taking an SGLT2 inhibitor, which has also been found to cause DKA, it is very likely you have Type 1 Diabetes or LADA rather than Type 2 Diabetes as people with Type 2 usually don't get DKA.

Years ago, it was hoped that starting insulin treatment very early in people at risk for autoimmune diabetes might lessen the immune system attack on the beta cells and help them survive longer, but this was not borne out by research conducted in children with the genes associated with Type 1 Diabetes. So there is no urgent need to start insulin if you have LADA and can keep your blood sugars in the normal range with diet.

Nevertheless, there evidence that people with Type 2 Diabetes, improve their long-term outcomes if they start insulin as soon as blood sugars become hard to control with diet. Since LADA combines genetic feature of both Type 1 and Type 2 diabetes, it is possible that using insulin early may still benefit people with LADA even if it doesn't stop the progression of the underlying autoimmune attack. In addition, new treatments are under development that may rescue the beta cells of people with LADA. Since you may need to still have some living beta cells to benefit from them, it is best to do what you can to preserve the cells you have left by keeping your blood sugar low enough to avoid killing them through glucose toxicity.

If there is any chance that you may have LADA, you should insist that your doctor run the appropriate tests and, if possible, refer you to an endocrinologist who is familiar with the condition.

Indicators that You May have LADA

❖ **A Family History of Type 1 Diabetes**. There is a genetic tendency toward developing autoimmune diabetes, so if you have a close family member who has autoimmune diabetes, it is more likely that you share that same genetic makeup and the same tendency toward developing autoimmune diabetes.

❖ **The Presence of Other Autoimmune Conditions**. If you already have another autoimmune condition like Rheumatoid Arthritis or Autoimmune Thyroid Disease it is more likely that your diabetes is also caused by an autoimmune attack. If this is the case, you may also be overweight or even obese due to these other conditions when you develop LADA. Since doctors assume that obese patients must have Type 2 Diabetes, they may not do the tests needed to determine if your diabetes is caused by autoimmunity.

❖ **Normal or Near Normal Weight Coupled with Very High Blood Sugars**. Although some people of normal weight do occasionally develop Type 2 Diabetes, many thin people in their 30s or 40s who are initially told they have Type 2 Diabetes turn out to have LADA. So LADA should always be ruled out in a thin or normal weight person diagnosed with Type 2 Diabetes, especially if blood sugars are extremely high at the time of diagnosis or if blood sugars deteriorate rapidly. LADA should not be a concern for normal weight people diagnosed with prediabetes unless they have a family history of Type 1 Diabetes or other autoimmune conditions.

❖ **Failure to Respond to Oral Drugs**. People with LADA often see swift deterioration in their blood sugars in the months after a Type 2 misdiagnosis. If your blood sugars are getting worse despite taking oral drugs and cutting back on carbohydrates—treatments that are usually effective for people recently diagnosed with Type 2 Diabetes—you should demand that your doctor test you for LADA or send you to an endocrinologist who will do this.

Diagnosing LADA

The most common test for LADA is one that looks for **GAD antibodies**. GAD stands for "glutamic acid decarboxylase." However, a small number of people with autoimmune diabetes will not have GAD antibodies. Instead they will have **islet cell antibodies** and/or **tyrosine phosphatase antibodies**. So a lack of GAD antibodies does not entirely rule out LADA. Antibody tests may come back normal if your symptoms began very recently and should be repeated a few months later if other symptoms still suggest LADA.

If you aren't already injecting insulin, an alternative way of testing for LADA is to test your fasting insulin level. A very low level is suggestive of LADA rather than Type 2 Diabetes. If you are injecting insulin, you will need a fasting C-peptide test to learn whether or not your beta cells are still making any insulin. C-peptide is only produced when your beta cells secrete insulin. Injected insulin does not provide any C-peptide. The C-peptide test is a crude, fairly inaccurate test that tells you only whether you are making normal, abnormally low, or abnormally high amounts of insulin. Changes in C-peptide values from test to test are not significant unless they are very large.

An extremely low C-peptide test result suggests that your beta cells have stopped making insulin, possibly because they are dead. C-peptide tests of people recently diagnosed with Type 2 Diabetes usually show normal or even high levels of C-peptide. This remains true for years after diagnosis, unless they allow their blood sugars to persist at levels high enough to kill off their remaining beta cells. So an extremely low C-peptide level, when it occurs along with the other symptoms described above, is suggestive of LADA, though that test result should be confirmed with antibody tests.

Treatment for LADA

People with LADA typically progress to a form of diabetes very similar to Type 1 over a period of roughly five years after diagnosis, though, as is so often the case, individual cases can vary considerably. I have heard from people diagnosed with LADA who did not become fully insulin dependent even eight years after diagnosis. But once a person progresses to full autoimmune diabetes, they need the same treatment given to people with Type 1 Diabetes. Most insurance plans will consider them eligible for insulin pumps, too, which many people find very helpful for achieving tight blood sugar control.

If you have LADA you should try to see an endocrinologist who specializes in treating Type 1 Diabetes. That kind of doctor can prescribe an up-to-date insulin regimen consisting of basal and fast-acting insulin, do the paperwork needed to qualify you for a pump if you choose to use one, and get you the intensive diabetes education given to people with Type 1 Diabetes.

MODY

A different kind of diabetes, which can be mistaken for either Type 2 or Type 1 Diabetes, is **Maturity Onset Diabetes of the Young** usually referred to as **MODY**. This term actually refers to several different, unrelated forms of diabetes that have in common only that they are genetic in origin and that they are **monogenic**. This means a person needs to inherit only a single defective gene to develop the disorder.

Most of the defective genes that cause the various forms of MODY cause the beta cells to fail to secrete insulin. In MODY-1 and MODY-3, this failure stops the secretion of insulin at meal-times, though fasting insulin may still be secreted. The gene found in the most common form of MODY, MODY-2, raises fasting blood sugar while not affecting post-meal insulin secretion. It is believed that some form of MODY may affect up to 5% of all people diagnosed with either Type 1 and Type 2 Diabetes. The most common forms are MODY-1, MODY-2, and MODY-3. The rest are very rare. MODY-4 has only been detected in a single family, MODY-6 in three.

Recent Research Has Changed Our Understanding of MODY

Until a decade ago, the commoner forms of MODY were thought only to affect people under the age of 25. However, genetic studies in which family members of people diagnosed with MODY were given genetic testing discovered that people carrying MODY genes can develop full-fledged diabetes as late as age 55. In addition, these studies found that quite a few people carrying MODY genes had been misdiagnosed as having Type 1 or Type 2 Diabetes, depending on the age of onset and severity of their case.

A study of the age of onset of MODY-3, one of the more common form of MODY, found that 65% of those diagnosed were diagnosed by age 25 and 100% by age 50. So more than one third of all people with this kind of diabetes do not have symptoms severe enough to lead to a diagnosis until middle age.

Because MODY is monogenic, doctors will usually rule it out if you don't have one parent diagnosed with diabetes. But recent research has also discovered that people carrying MODY genes sometimes have blood sugar problems so mild that they escape diagnosis. So while it is true that a person with MODY usually inherits the gene from a parent who carries the MODY gene, the fact that your parent was *not* diagnosed with diabetes does not rule out the possibility that you have it, especially if other people in your family have been diagnosed with a milder form of Type 1 Diabetes, or with Type 2 Diabetes that came on when they were at a normal or near normal weight, or even, in some cases, with impaired fasting glucose or impaired glucose tolerance.

MODY genes may express less strongly if you inherited the gene from your father. That is because, if the MODY gene comes from your mother, she will have had gestational diabetes during pregnancy. Exposure to high blood sugars during pregnancy makes the gene express more strongly in her offspring.

How Do You Get Diagnosed with MODY?

Unfortunately, the only way to get a definitive diagnosis it to take expensive genetic tests, which may still be inconclusive since Athena Diagnostics, the company that provides this testing, reports that their six gene tests only identify 85% of the cases of MODY found in the United States population.

Many health insurers won't pay for these genetic tests, so if you can't get MODY testing, you may have to approach a diagnosis by looking at your family history, your personal history, your weight history, and indications of how insulin resistant you are.

Below are some factors that suggest that it is possible you have MODY. *In all cases MODY should only be considered if you or your family members do not test positive for any of the antibodies diagnostic of autoimmune diabetes.* Autoimmune diabetes is *far* more common than any form of MODY.

❖ If you were diagnosed with diabetes when you were younger than 30 no matter what your weight or if you were diagnosed younger than 45 and weren't overweight you may have MODY, as long as tests show you have a normal fasting C-peptide level and no markers of autoimmune disease. Fifteen percent of subjects in one study given gene analyses who fit these criteria turned out to have MODY-1 or MODY-3.

❖ If you have a history of gestational diabetes that occurred when you began the pregnancy at a normal weight.

❖ If you have close relatives who had adult onset diabetes who were of normal weight.

❖ If taking drugs that improve insulin resistance like metformin or Actos don't make any difference in your blood sugar or A1c.

❖ If, without taking any diabetes drugs, you have glucose in your urine when your blood sugar has not risen higher than 160 mg/dl after a meal, especially if there is a history of kidney disease in your family. People with MODY-1, -3, and -5 sometimes have subtle or even serious kidney malformations that cause them to spill glucose in their urine at relatively low blood sugars.

❖ If you have a very strong response to an insulin-stimulating drug. People with MODY-1 or -3 may see intense blood sugar drops after taking as little as ¼ of the smallest dose of a sulfonylurea or meglitinide drug.

❖ If you have very low cardiac-specific CRP. A study published in 2010 found that People with MODY-3 have very low cs-CRP.

❖ If your fasting blood sugar has always been higher than normal and does not come down when you take metformin or basal insulin. This would point to MODY-2, which only raises fasting blood sugar.

Indications You Do *Not* Have MODY

MODY is fairly rare. To avoid wasting your money on expensive testing, it's important to know that the following symptoms make it very *unlikely* you have any form of MODY.

❖ High fasting insulin or C-peptide level. High levels of insulin present when blood sugars are higher than normal suggest that you are insulin resistant, not insulin deficient. People with MODY are usually very sensitive to insulin.

❖ Sudden onset of abnormal blood sugars that deteriorate swiftly. People with MODY are born with MODY and will have at least slightly abnormal blood sugars all their lives. Their blood sugars may become worse with increasing age, pregnancy, or other physiological stressors, but in general the progress is gradual. The sudden onset of abnormal blood sugar or a blood sugar that deteriorates dramatically over a brief period is more likely to point to the adult-onset form of autoimmune diabetes called LADA.

❖ Use of typical insulin doses. If you are using a standard sized dose of insulin, you aren't likely to have one of the common forms of MODY. People with these forms of MODY typically need only the very small insulin doses that people with Type 1 use only during the early "honeymoon" stage of their condition—two or three units to cover a high carbohydrate meal. In addition, because there is often intact basal insulin secretion, a person with MODY may need very little injected basal insulin. If you are using over 20 units a day of basal insulin or injecting more than 7 units of fast-acting insulin to cover a high carbohydrate meal you are unlikely to have any of the commoner forms of MODY.

Treating MODY

Most forms of MODY are very much like Type 2 Diabetes in how they affect your body. Elevated blood sugars injure you slowly over many years, causing neuropathy, retinopathy, heart disease and the other ugly complications of diabetes.

In families who carry genes for forms of MODY considered "mild" it is quite common to see many people dying of heart attacks before the age of 60, thanks to a lifetime of exposure to *prediabetic* blood sugars that elude diagnosis. This makes it essential that people with any form of MODY strive for the same normal blood sugars recommended for those diagnosed with more common forms of diabetes.

The recommended treatment for MODY depends on the severity of the diabetes. Some people with MODY can maintain normal blood sugar levels by restricting carbohydrates. Others may be treated with low doses of an insulin-stimulating drug or small doses of insulin.

Doctors assume you'd prefer a pill to shots, so they often suggest sulfonylurea drugs rather than insulin. But the insulin-stimulating drugs that are prescribed for people diagnosed with MODY may cause the hunger and weight gain typical of these drugs. In addition, as we discussed earlier, the sulfonylurea drugs available in the United States promote heart disease. Repaglinide is the only safe drug available to people with MODY in the United States, but it must be used very carefully, as over time it can cause hypos. Gliclazide is the safe drug recommended for people with MODY in the rest of the world.

The advantage of using an insulin-stimulating drug is that when your body secretes its own insulin, it also produces C-peptide. C-peptide was long believed to be inert, but recent research has found that, in fact, it plays an important part in preventing vascular complications. Injecting insulin may shut down native insulin production of C-peptide, so a person with MODY who injects insulin may be slightly more prone to developing microvascular complications.

But many people with MODY diabetes find that using very low doses of insulin at meal times gives them better control, less hunger, and avoids hypos. People with MODY who cut back on carbs can often get by using very small doses—2 or 3 units per meal.

If you suspect you have MODY and your doctor wants you to start insulin or an insulin stimulating drug, be sure to start at a very low dose. The doses appropriate for Type 2 may cause dramatic hypos in people with MODY, because the starting dose of either an insulin-stimulating drug or insulin appropriate for an insulin-resistant person with Type 2 Diabetes may be two to ten times higher than the dose that works well for a person with MODY.

When starting insulin, start with one unit and work up to the appropriate dose. Many people with MODY may do well with as little as 4-12 units a day. A typical Type 2 may use anywhere from 30 to 100 units. If using insulin stimulating pills, start with ¼ of a pill and test blood sugar frequently to check for hypos.

If you suspect you have MODY diabetes and are of childbearing age, and if there is a strong history of diabetes in your spouse's family, consider genetic testing. A child who inherits two copies of the same MODY gene will be born with a severe form of diabetes, though given the rarity of MODY the chances of this occurring are extremely low. The chances are higher if you and your spouse share the same ethnic heritage.

Should You Ignore MODY-2?

After a study was published in 2015 that documented that people with MODY-2 do not get the classic diabetic complications—retinopathy, neuropathy, and kidney disease—endocrinologists have started to advise people diagnosed with MODY-2 that they do not need to do anything to control their abnormally high blood sugars.

However, I have heard from quite a few people who have been diagnosed with MODY-2 whose families are full of people who died of heart attacks when they were under 60 years old. Since heart attacks are not considered by most doctors to be a diabetic complication, the research dismissing the connection between MODY-2 and diabetic complications did not examine that association. This suggests that people with MODY-2 should, like everyone else, take steps to lower their post-meal blood sugars.

Doctors tell people with MODY-2 that this is not possible, probably because none of the commonly prescribed diabetes drugs help people with MODY. However, I have also heard from several people with MODY-2 diagnoses who report that lowering their carbohydrate intake at meals *has* lowered their fasting blood sugar significantly. They also find it controls their post-meal blood sugar spikes. If you have MODY-2 there is no harm in testing whether lowering carbohydrates lowers your post-meal blood sugars, since it is high post-meal blood sugars that raise the risk of developing heart disease.

Do It Yourself MODY Testing

If you suspect you have MODY but can't get your insurer to pay for genetic testing there are three simple tests that may help you decide if it might be worth it to pay for the tests yourself.

The Renal Threshold Test for MODY-3

People with MODY-3 often have an abnormally low renal threshold for glucose. This means they will spill glucose into urine at abnormally low blood sugar levels. In most people glucose appears in urine when blood sugar reaches 160-180 mg/dl. However, people with MODY-3 may find glucose in their urine when their blood sugar has only risen to 140 mg/dl.

You can test your own renal threshold by buying the urine test strips for glucose carried by most pharmacies. Test your urine one, two, and three hours after eating a meal that did not raise your one hour blood sugar over 150 mg/dl. If you have other symptoms characteristic of MODY and see glucose in your urine when your blood sugar did not go higher than 150 mg/dl, it is more likely that you do, in fact, have MODY-3. (This test will not work if you are taking a SGLT2 drug like Invokana or Jardiance that lowers the renal threshold for glucose.)

People with MODY-3 are also more likely to develop kidney disease, so if you find a low renal threshold, be sure your doctor monitors your kidney health. If there is a family history of kidney disease, be sure to have your kidneys evaluated by a nephrologist.

Sulfonylurea Sensitivity Test

You will need your doctor's help to perform this test. Explain that you believe you may have MODY and that people with MODY are extremely sensitive to sulfonylurea drugs. Then ask your doctor to prescribe the very smallest size dose available of any cheap generic sulfonylurea drug, for example, glyburide or glimepiride.

Divide the pill into quarters using a sharp knife or a pill cutter. Be sure you have high carbohydrate foods on hand in case you have a strong response to the drug, as a strong response can cause long-lasting hypos. Do not take any basal insulin. Take one quarter of the tablet and eat a meal containing at least 30 grams of carbohydrates. Test your blood sugar throughout the day. If your blood sugar stays flat or drops over the next eight hours, you are very sensitive to insulin stimulation in a way that suggests you may indeed have MODY-1 or -3. If your blood sugar drops below 85 mg/dl eat high carbohydrate food every few hours, as it may take up to eight hours until the drug stops affecting your blood sugars. You may also find yourself ravenously hungry during the whole time the drug is active.

Report your experience to your doctor. He should find it unusual, as people with Type 2 can usually take anywhere from two to eight times as high a dose of a sulfonylurea drug before seeing a significant drop in blood sugar.

Hs-CRP Testing

If you suspect that you have MODY-3, a low hs-CRP test result may be diagnostic. People with MODY-3 have an average hs-CRP test result or 0.20 mg/1 with a range of 0.03 to 1.14 mg/1. The researchers who discovered this suggest that testing CRP may provide a cheap and effective screening test MODY-3 as it appears to identify 80% of people diagnosed with Type 2 diabetes who actually have it. However, the rest of the commoner forms of MODY do not produce low hs-CRP results.

Insulin Sensitive Type 2 Diabetes

There is another possibility to consider if you have many of the symptoms described above but do not appear to have MODY.

There are other unidentified genetic defects, besides the ones that are defined as MODY, that cause *insulin sensitive* forms of Type 2 Diabetes. Though the genes at fault may be different than those causing MODY, the clinical manifestations may be the same: high blood sugars along with a lack of obesity, the development of gestational diabetes at a normal weight, and normal or high sensitivity to injected insulin.

All these suggest that your problem is a secretory defect rather than insulin resistance. For some reason, your beta cells are not secreting insulin when blood sugars start to rise. The treatment options for these kinds of Type 2 Diabetes are similar to the treatment options used for MODY: Insulin after meals, possibly combined with very low dose basal insulin or else insulin stimulating drugs at low doses.

But whatever the cause for your diabetes, the fundamental principle in treating it doesn't change. If you keep your blood sugar at normal levels, you should be able to avoid complications, and the best way to do that is to go easy on the carbohydrates and use only those drugs that have been proven to be safe.

Chapter Fourteen
Working with Doctors and Hospitals

Doctors who keep up-to-date with the latest diabetes and dietary research can help you avoid a future filled with amputations, failing vision, and dialysis.

Not all doctors do keep up. In fact, quite a few of the doctors in practice today got their only formal training in diabetes care during their residencies decades ago, and the only "diabetes education" they've gotten since then has been provided by drug company representatives. This drug company "education" is nothing more than promotion for whatever are the newest, most expensive drugs available for treating diabetes. Sadly, because the dietary approach we suggest in these pages does not enrich any company, no salespeople or high profile doctors on corporate payrolls promote it to doctors.

Many conscientious but overworked doctors get their information about new diabetes treatments from professional newsletters that report on the latest advances in patient care. But these too, tend to be heavily influenced by drug company press releases and supported by drug company advertising.

And because doctors in general practice must keep up with many dozens of serious diseases besides diabetes, doctors who are very good at treating some conditions may not be as good at treating others that haven't captured their interest. Unfortunately, diabetes often falls into the latter category. So you will have to ask some hard questions to determine if a doctor you are seeing is capable of being an ally who can help you master your diabetes.

Do You Have a Good Doctor?

Below you will find a list of questions you can use to determine this. Use them to ensure that your doctor is a partner, not an obstacle, in your quest for normal health.

Does Your Doctor Support You in Your Efforts to Attain Normal Blood Sugars?

Be wary of any doctor who dismisses your concern about an abnormal blood sugar test because he thinks it isn't abnormal enough.

If your fasting blood sugar is over 110 mg/dl, or your post-meal blood sugars are routinely over 150 mg/dl two hours after eating, and your doctor tells you that this is normal or nothing to worry about, they are making it clear they are not aware of what mainstream medical practitioners now know about the impact of prediabetes. The same is true if your A1c is over 6.5% and your doctor discourages you from improving it. A doctor who considers elevated blood sugars "nothing to worry about" is likely to put roadblocks in the way of your getting better control or may lull you into a false sense of security.

Some particularly toxic doctors, who have been swayed by misinterpretation of the ACCORD data we discussed in Chapter Four, may even take away your prescriptions for the safe drugs that got your A1c down below 6.5% because they still believe that it is dangerous to lower A1c below that level.

You should not have to wait until you've lost all feeling in your toes, had your first retinal hemorrhage, or have lab tests showing protein in your urine to have your doctor start taking your blood sugar seriously.

Does Your Doctor Order Appropriate Tests?

If your doctor believes you only need a fasting plasma glucose test or A1c test to rule out diabetes and ignores it when you report experiencing high blood sugars after meals—especially readings over 200 mg/dl—you may be on the way to developing any of the diabetic complications that start at officially "prediabetic" levels.

The ADA used to warn doctors that the A1c test was not a valid test for diagnosing diabetes because the A1c can return deceptively low values if a person is anemic or has certain genetic red blood cell variants. Their recent switch to endorsing the A1c test to screen for diabetes ignores a wealth of research that documents that the A1c test does a poor job of diagnosing individuals. The switch was probably made because the cheap A1c test saves insurance plans money. If your doctor insists you only need an A1c test and ignores post-meal readings, beware.

Once you have been diagnosed with diabetes, your doctor should offer you an A1c test at least two times a year and discuss the test results with you. If possible, ask that the A1c test be done at a lab, since research has found that many of the in-office tests sold to doctors aren't very accurate. Unfortunately, because doctors can bill insurers for them, these inaccurate in-office tests have become increasingly common.

If your A1c is over 6.5%, your doctor should work with you to get your A1c under the 6.5% level recommended by the American Association of Clinical Endocrinologists. If you prod him, your doctor should be willing to help you get it under 6%. If your doctor warns you that lowering A1c below 6.5% is dangerous, *when you are not using Actos or Avandia or experiencing frequent hypos,* find another doctor.

A good doctor should also annually test your urinary microalbumin, which is a measure of kidney health. If you are on medications, your doctor should also order liver enzyme tests periodically to make sure that you aren't being injured by the drugs you are taking. If you are on metformin, you should have your B-12 levels checked every few years.

You will also know that your doctor is knowledgeable about diabetes if he tests the pulses in your ankles to check the quality of your circulation and uses a filament or tuning fork to test the nerves in your feet. Your doctor should also refer you to an ophthalmologist for an eye exam each year. An ophthalmologist is a physician who specializes in the treatment of the eyes and is far more highly trained than the optometrists who do most eye exams.

If your doctor finds anything in your test results suggestive of early diabetic complications, they should urge you to lower your blood sugars and work with you to find a safe drug regimen that will supplement the changes you make in your diet.

Does Your Doctor Prescribe Drugs Appropriately?

The practice recommendations published by the ultra-conservative American Diabetes Association state that metformin should be the first drug that doctors prescribe to a patient with Type 2 Diabetes. That's because metformin reduces insulin resistance and has a long safety record. Competent doctors should also know that the ER (extended release) form of metformin does not cause as much stomach distress as the plain form. The cost of the ER version of the drug is the same as that of the regular so there is no reason not to prescribe the ER form.

Unfortunately, old fashioned doctors are also still prescribing sulfonylurea drugs as the first drug they give their diabetic patients, unaware that these drugs almost always cause hunger that results in weight gain, which increases insulin resistance and makes a heart attack more likely.

Other doctors give newly diagnosed patients whatever is the newest, most heavily marketed, expensive diabetes drug—often without understanding exactly what it is that these new drugs do. Be cautious about a doctor who starts you on Januvia, Victoza, Saxenda, Invokana, or Jardiance before trying a course of plain metformin and advising you to cut back on your carbohydrates. None of the newer patented diabetes drugs lowers insulin resistance and they often don't do a good job of lowering blood sugar.

Be wary of doctors who prescribe combo drugs containing fixed doses of metformin and expensive new patented drugs. As we explained in Chapter Nine, you may not be able to adjust your dose of metformin up to the level where it becomes effective without raising the dose of the other drug to where it causes serious side effects.

If your doctor does prescribe a brand new drug that has only been on the market for a short time, demand to know why you aren't being given some older drug with a longer track record. Be wary if you are told the new drug has fewer side effects, since the real side effect profile of a new drug can't be known until it has been on the market for several years.

Does Your Doctor Suggest Insulin When Oral Drugs Aren't Normalizing Blood Sugar?

If you have tried two or three oral medications and are still seeing high blood sugars, your doctor should suggest that you use insulin to get your blood sugars into the safe zone.

Insulin works, and modern insulins are much easier to use than those available in the past. If you have Type 2 Diabetes and your fasting blood sugar is still higher than 125 mg/dl with oral medications, your doctor should suggest a basal insulin like Lantus or Levemir if you have health insurance that will cover it at a cost you can afford. If you don't, ask your doctor if you can use one of the cheaper regular human insulins.

If using a basal insulin does not allow you to keep your post-meal blood sugars under 200 mg/dl when eating high carbohydrate meals, your doctor should be willing to refer you to an endocrinologist who can start you on meal-time insulin.

If You Are Not Getting Results or Are Having Troubling Side Effects Your Doctor Should Stop a Medication

One of the most worrisome things I observe in people posting on the web is the number of people who are experiencing what are known to be the dangerous side effects of commonly prescribed medications, whose doctors tell them to keep on taking them. Such side effects include muscle pain from statins, severe water retention with Actos or pain and vomiting with Byetta or Victoza. The first two symptoms can lead to permanent organ damage. The latter may point to pancreatitis.

Even worse, many patients report being put on expensive drugs that don't do much for their blood sugars and being told to keep taking them to "preserve their beta cells." If an expensive drug is not improving your blood sugar, there is no reason to take it. No drug will preserve or rejuvenate your beta cells if you are running blood sugars in the range that causes the glucotoxicity that kills them.

Does Your Doctor Know That Cutting Carbohydrates Is Safe and Effective?

Though there has been some improvement over the past decade in how open doctors are to the idea of cutting carbs to lower blood sugar, there are still many doctors telling people with diabetes to eat low fat/high carbohydrate diets, as if it were fat, rather than carbohydrates that raises blood sugar. Some even warn patients that the low carbo-hydrate diet is dangerous, though even the American Diabetes Asso-ciation revised its practice recommendations in 2008 to state that low carbohydrate diets are safe for people with diabetes.

Though they may not be enthusiastic about low carbohydrate diet-ing, your doctors should be aware that eliminating as much carbohy-drate from your diet as possible and replacing that carbohydrate with fat is a safe and effective way to lower blood sugars. Your doctor should also know that the evidence now points to it being dietary car-bohydrate that worsens lipids, not fat, and that eating a low fat diet doesn't prevent heart disease.

Is Your Doctor's Staff Reasonable and Accessible?

Because family doctors are so overburdened, many of them have set up their practices so you don't deal with them directly but must talk to staff members when routine matters come up. These staff members may be highly trained nurse practitioners as competent as the doctor when it comes to handling routine requests or they may be LPN nurses with only a year of education beyond high school who never-theless believe themselves competent to screen your call, though they may not understand what you tell them well enough to pass on an accurate message to the doctor.

It is very important to find a practice where the staff members you have to deal with are helpful, friendly, and, most importantly, intelli-gent enough to be able to convey your concerns to your doctor with-out garbling them. If your doctor refers all patients to a "diabetes nurse" for day-to-day case management, this is even more important. No matter how good your doctor is, you won't get good care if you have to go through a diabetes nurse who considers your call with a question about a high blood sugar frivolous or who believes that any A1c below 7.0% is "great control" no matter what kinds of numbers you are seeing after meals.

If your doctor expects a nurse to help you adjust your insulin doses, ask what that nurse's training has been. Ideally you'd like them to be a

Certified Diabetes Educator. Find out, too, how long it has been since they've updated their training. There are a lot of "diabetes nurses" out there who are still treating patients with insulin regimens from twenty years ago—the kind that avoid hypos by allowing your blood sugar to rise dangerously high or force you to eat a lot of carbohydrates to keep from going low.

What to Expect of a Good Doctor

Even with the very best doctor you are going to have to do a lot of the work of managing your diabetes yourself. Diabetes is the ultimate "do it yourself" condition. Keep up with the diabetes news by tuning into web discussion groups, blogs, or online newsletters like *Diabetes in Control*. When you've done all you can on your own, ask your doctor to help you evaluate the information you have found. A good doctor should:

❖ Help you try out a new diabetes treatment you've heard about or explain clearly why it isn't appropriate for you.

❖ Order appropriate tests after explaining to you what questions the tests can answer.

❖ Give you your actual test results, not a summary, and explain to you what these test results mean, answering any questions you may have about the test result.

❖ Give you a copy of your lab test results when you ask for them. You have a right to your test results and should always ask to have a copy made for you before you leave the office. Keep these test results in a file, as you may need to refer to them in the future if you change doctors. When doctors transfer records they often do not send your old lab tests.

❖ Refer you to an appropriate specialist if something comes up that is not in their area of competence—and be honest about what that area of competence includes.

❖ If you don't have insurance or are in financial difficulty, explain to you how to sign up for drug company or state programs to help you get the drugs you need to preserve your health. The office staff should also be willing to fill in any necessary paperwork you need for insurance approvals or hardship drug support programs.

Diabetes at the Hospital or Nursing Home

If you have diabetes and are forced to go to a hospital, emergency room, or nursing home for any reason at all, you may find yourself plunged into a situation where well-intentioned but ignorant medical professionals do all they can to destroy your blood sugar control.

Because none of us know when we may be the victim of an accident or disease, every person with diabetes should prepare a "Medical Instruction Letter" signed by their primary care doctor or endocrinologist. This letter should describe in detail the diet and medications you should be given if you are hospitalized or put into a nursing home.

Hospitals and nursing homes still force patients with diabetes to eat the discredited low fat/high carbohydrate diet. They often use outdated "sliding scale" insulin dosing schemes, which guarantee that patients will experience very high post-meal blood sugars. I have heard several stories about people put in nursing homes who had maintained excellent blood sugars before being institutionalized but were forced by the nursing home staff to eat very high carbohydrate meals and forbidden to set their own insulin doses even though they were mentally competent. The outdated care they received ruined their blood sugar control and in some cases contributed to their deaths.

Your Own Doctor No Longer Treats You at the Hospital

Over the past decade many hospitals have moved from the system where your own doctor visited you and dictated your treatment to a new system where a stranger called a "hospitalist" has complete control over your fate while you are hospitalized. The hospitalist is a doctor who treats you only while you are in the hospital and has no idea what treatment your regular doctor has prescribed for you. They may not even have access to your medical records. They specialize in critical care and are not likely to have been trained in the daily treatment of diabetes. If you are on insulin, they may forbid you to administer your own shots and put you at the mercy of nurses who use old-fashioned, generic ways of dosing. Even worse, a doctor at the hospital who sees the word "diabetes" on your chart may assume you have heart disease and order expensive tests completely unrelated to the reason that you went to the hospital, simply because they assume that because you have diabetes *any* symptom you have—including those resulting from accidents—must be a diabetic complication.

Don't Expect Anything You Say in the Hospital to Be Respected

Once you are signed into a hospital or nursing home, nothing you say will have any effect on your treatment, because the hospital and nursing home culture is one where only "Doctor's Orders" prevail.

If the hospitalist assigned your care believes that you should be eating a high carb/low fat diet, that's what you will be served. If they believe you should be given insulin on a sliding scale, that's what you'll be given. The only option you have in this situation is to sign out of the hospital with the words "against medical advice" put into your medical records. This is not feasible if you are in the hospital because of an accident or surgery.

Protect Yourself with a Doctor's Letter

Protect yourself with a letter that you draw up before you need it. You must have it put on your doctor's stationary and signed by your regular doctor. This letter should be entered into your medical records at your local hospital. You should carry a copy to the hospital or have your next of kin bring it to the hospital as soon as you are admitted.

Here's what to include in your hospital letter:

❖ Have your doctor state that you are a highly compliant patient whose diabetes control is excellent and/or exemplary. State your A1c if it is under 6%.

❖ Have the doctor describe the diet that you should be placed on should you be hospitalized. If you are eating a low carbohydrate diet, it is not enough to say you are eating a "carbohydrate restricted" diet. My local hospital feeds people with diabetes what they describe as a "Carbohydrate Restricted Diabetes Diet." It provides 50 grams of carbohydrate per meal and no fat. If you are put on this diet, the nutrition department will refuse to serve you any foods containing fat. In addition, the amount of protein in the meals they provide for people with diabetes is very low, which would be a serious concern if you were in the hospital for surgery or healing from a wound.

❖ To avoid being put on this kind of dangerous "diabetes diet," you must have your doctor specify that you should be given a diet whose *percentage* of fat, protein, and carbohydrate per meal is specified.

❖ Have the doctor specify that if you are conscious you should be in charge of administering your own insulin and that you should be allowed to do your own blood sugar testing using your own equipment. Otherwise you may have your insulin and blood testing supplies removed at admission.

❖ If you are not conscious, you will be at the mercy of your local hospital staff. Discuss this problem with your doctor in advance and ask for suggestions as to how it can be dealt with.

That's it for now. I hope you have found this book useful. If you use the techniques you find here and find them helpful, do share what you've learned with others who might benefit from this knowledge. Working together we can ensure that people with diabetes have the same chance for normal, healthy life as everyone else.

—Jenny Ruhl

Appendix A
Convert Mg/dl to Mmol/L

Blood Sugar in mg/dl	Blood Sugar in mmol/L
20	1.1
50	2.8
60	3.3
70	3.9
85	4.7
90	5.0
100	5.5
108	6.0
110	6.1
120	6.6
125	6.9
140	7.8
150	8.3
180	10.0
200	11.1
250	13.9
500	27.7

Table 6. Blood Sugar Equivalents: mg/dl to mmol/L

This table uses the accurate conversion factor of 18.05. However, you will often see slightly different values given for equivalents as many people round the conversion factor down by 18. The very small difference this produces is not significant when using these numbers to set blood sugar targets.

Appendix B

What Can You Eat When You Are Cutting the Carbs?

Here are some foods that should be kind to your blood sugar, which have been suggested by people posting on web diet and diabetes support groups. Some helpful recipes can also be found at: http://bloodsugar101.com/recipes.php.

❖ **Pancakes**. Whey Protein powder can be cooked up to make pancakes as can cottage cheese. Add some fresh strawberries, blueberries, or raspberries and some sugar free Maple Syrup and you've got a delicious breakfast. Frozen berries work very well, too.

❖ **Fauxtatoes.** A great substitute for mashed potatoes can be made by steaming or boiling cauliflower and pureeing it in a food processor with some cream or half and half, butter and salt. The result tastes much more like mashed potatoes than cauliflower.

❖ **Rolls.** Bake delicious rolls very similar to popovers using the "Magic Rolls" recipe from the Eades' *Low Carb Comfort Food Cookbook*. Make extra and freeze in a plastic bag. If you can't handle gluten, try making "oopsies," egg and cream cheese rolls you'll find described on the **lowcarbfriends.com** discussion forum.

❖ **Veggies.** Here's a list of some healthy very low carbohydrate vegetables you should eat as much as possible: mesclun mix, green beans, artichokes, avocado, asparagus, boston lettuce, broccoli, brussels sprouts, cabbage, cauliflower, collard greens, cucumbers, eggplant, kale, olives, red lettuce, romaine lettuce, spaghetti squash, spinach, swiss chard, yellow summer squash, zucchini. The lower your carbohydrate intake, the better they will taste. Fresh peppers and tomatoes work for most people, too, though they both contain some carbohydrate.

❖ **Soup.** Make homemade soups with broth, meat, and the vegetables listed above. Add a tablespoon of salsa or curry to add flavor and variety. Cream and cheese soups are also delicious, especially if you add pureed cauliflower or broccoli instead of flour to thicken them.

❖ **Pasta.** Instead of using pasta with its over 50 grams of carbohydrate per tiny two ounce serving, pour your pasta sauces over lightly steamed zucchini strips you make with a vegetable peeler or spirilizer. Another alternative is spaghetti squash. Shiritake noodles, which contain a fiber called glucomannan, are also very low in carbohydrate, though they are one of those foods people either love or hate. Avoid pastas containing soy as soy can be hard on your thyroid gland.

❖ **Sugar Substitutes.** Though there is conflicting information about the usefulness of sugar substitutes for weight loss, if your goal is to control your blood sugar, they work very well. Splenda and stevia are safe, though stevia becomes bitter if you bake with it. A mixture of Splenda and erythritol powder works well for baked goods, though erythritol on its own does not do a good job of sweetening hot drinks. When baking, instead of Splenda powder, use DaVinci sugar free syrups for sweetening. Splenda powder contains maltodextrin, a sugar. In large portions, the carbohydrates in Splenda powder can add up. The DaVinci sugar free syrups contain no added sugars. These can be ordered online. When baking, use a direct substitution: one teaspoon of sugar free syrup for one teaspoon of sugar. This works well for cheesecakes and custards.

❖ **Cookies.** You can make delicious very low carbohydrate macaroons with recipes you can find searching online. You can also make cookies using almonds ground very fine, but do not use almond flour if you are having trouble losing weight as it is very high in calories.

❖ **Snack Food.** Sunflower seeds in the shell make a good "finger food" snack. They are very low in carbohydrates and can take the place of chips while watching the game, etc. You can make snack chips by microwaving pepperoni slices or small pieces of cheese on parchment paper.

❖ **Candy.** Low carb cream cheese fudge or fudge made by cooling coconut oil makes a nice chocolate candy treat. You can find recipes for these online.

❖ **Pizza.** When it's pizza time, get a meat/veggie combo and just eat the toppings. Some people make "meatza" using a thin lining of pepperoni as the bottom crust when they make pizza at home.

❖ **Chinese Restaurants.** Try hot and sour soup, teriyaki strips, crispy duck, ginger chicken, or beef with string beans, and black bean sauce dishes as they are less likely to have sugary sauces. Ask for spareribs without any extra sauce. There are carbohydrates in all of these, so make this a rare treat.

❖ **Thai restaurants**. Most of Thai dishes served in American Thai restaurants are drenched in sugar. The combination of sugar and starch in Pad Thai means a very small serving can easily contain more than 110 grams of carbohydrate. Curries may also be thickened with rice powder. Stick with meat on skewers, duck and seafood dishes served without noodles or rice, or visit these restaurants on a day when you are eating off-plan.

❖ **Other Restaurants** Besides the obvious "chunk o' meat" entrees try the steak "bistro" salads or Caesar salads with grilled chicken or shrimp (not breaded and fried!). Avoid salads where you can't add the dressing yourself, as some chains call bits of lettuce and meat drenched in sugar "salad." Stick with blue cheese, parmesan peppercorn, ranch, oil and vinegar, or classic Italian dressing. Many flavored vinaigrettes are full of sugar. Many Steak House chains sprinkle MSG on their steaks, which may improve flavor but leaves you ravenously hungry an hour later. Avoid those restaurants if you're trying to lose weight!

❖ **Nuts**. Almonds, walnuts, and pecans are low in carbohydrates and full of healthy oils. You can heat them on a cookie sheet for a few minutes with a coating of DaVinci flavored syrup to make them into a fancy treat.

❖ **Sinful Desserts**. Bake a low carbohydrate cheesecake. Use the Classic Philly 3 Step Cheesecake recipe. Substitute DaVinci sugar free syrup for the sugar and bake for a few minutes longer than usual. Instead of graham crackers, use a crushed nut crust made by chopping walnuts or almonds and pressing them into the pan.

❖ **Inventive Recipes.** You'll find many excellent low carb recipes at the web site, "Linda's Low Carb Menus and Recipes" which is found at **http://www.genaw.com/lowcarb**. Another good source for ideas is the collection of recipes that were originally posted on the old alt.support.diet.low-carb newsgroup, found online at: **http://www.camacdonald.com/lc/LowCarbohydrateCooking-Recipes.htm**. If you prefer a printed cookbook, Dana Carpender's book, *500 Low-Carb Recipes* is highly recommended.

Diabetes Drug Families

Class	Generic Name	Brand Name
	Drugs that lower Insulin Resistance	
Biguanides	Metformin	Glucophage, Glumetza
Thiazolidinedione	Rosiglitazone	Avandia
	Pioglitazone	Actos
	Insulin Stimulating Drugs	
Sulfonylureas	Glyburide	DiaBeta
	Gliclazide	Diamicron
	Glipizide	Glucotrol
	Glimepiride	Amaryl
Meglitinides	Repaglinide	Prandin
	Nateglinide	Starlix
	Incretin Drugs	
DPP-4 Inhibitors	Sitagliptin	Januvia
	Saxagliptin	Onglyza
	Linagliptin	Trajenta
	Alogliptin	Nesina
GLP-1 Agonists	Exenatide	Byetta, Bydureon
	Liraglutide	Victoza, Saxenda
	Albiglutide	Tanzeum
	Dulaglutide	Trulicity
	Lixisenatide	Lyxumia
	Urinary Excretion Drugs	
SGLT-2 Inhibitors	Canagliflozin	Invokana
	Dapagliflozin	Forxiga
	Empagliflozin	Jardiance
	Insulins	
Basal Insulin	Isophane Insulin (NPH)	Novolin N, Humulin N
	Insulin Glargine	Lantus, Toujeo
	Insulin Detemir	Levemir
	Insulin Degludec	Tresiba
Fast-Acting Insulin	Regular Human	Novolin R, Humulin R
	Insulin Lispro	Humalog
	Insulin Aspart	Novolog
	Insulin Glulisine	Apidra
Ultra Fast Insulin	Technosphere Insulin	Afrezza

References

Chapter One: Normal Blood Sugar

The Genetic Basis of Type 2 Diabetes Mellitus: Impaired Insulin Secretion Versus Impaired Insulin Sensitivity. John E. Gerich. *Endocrine Reviews,* 19 (4):491-503

Normal fasting plasma glucose levels and type 2 diabetes in young men. Tirosh A et al. *N Engl J Med,* 2005 Oct 6;353(14):1454-62

Is Reduced First-Phase Insulin Release the Earliest Detectable Abnormality in Individuals Destined to Develop Type 2 Diabetes? John E. Gerich. *Diabetes,* 51:S117-S121, 2002

What is Normal Glucose? – Continuous Glucose Monitoring Data from Healthy Subjects. Professor J.S. Christiansen. Presented at the Annual Meeting of the EASD, 9/13/06

Variation of Interstitial Glucose Measurements Assessed by Continuous Glucose Monitors in Healthy, Nondiabetic Individuals. Juvenile Diabetes Research Foundation Continuous Glucose Monitoring Study Group. *Diabetes Care,* June 2010 vol. 33 no. 6 1297-1299

Diagnosis and Classification of Diabetes Mellitus. American Diabetes Association. *Diabetes Care,* 27:S5-S10, 2004

Chapter Two: How Diabetes Develops

You can read the history of how the American Diabetes Association set the arbitrary blood sugar levels used to diagnose diabetes at: http://www.bloodsugar101.com/14046782.php

A1C: Does One Size Fit All? Robert M. Cohen. *Diabetes Care,* October 2007 vol. 30 no. 10 2756-2758

Six of Eight Hemoglobin A1c Point-of-Care Instruments Do Not Meet the General Accepted Analytical Performance Criteria. Erna Lenters-Westra1, et al. *Clinical Chemistry,* 56:44-52, 2010

The Natural History of Progression from Normal Glucose Tolerance to Type 2 Diabetes in the Baltimore Longitudinal Study of Aging. James B. Meigs et al. *Diabetes,* 52:1475-1484, 2003

Natural History of Insulin Sensitivity and Insulin Secretion in the Progression From Normal Glucose Tolerance to Impaired Fasting Glycemia and Impaired Glucose Tolerance: The Inter99 Study. Kristine Færch, et al. *Diabetes Care,* 32:439-444, 2009

Mode of Onset of Type 2 Diabetes from Normal or Impaired Glucose Tolerance. Ele Ferrannini et al. *Diabetes,* 53(1):160-5 2003

Prevalence of the Metabolic Syndrome Among US Adults: Findings from the Third National Health and Nutrition Examination Survey. Earl S. Ford et al. *JAMA,* 2002;287:356-359

Prevalence of Obesity, Diabetes, and Obesity-Related Health Risk Factors, 2001. Ali H. Mokdad et al. *JAMA,* 2003;289:76-79

Hyperglycemia and insulin resistance: possible mechanisms. Tomás E et al. *Ann N Y Acad Sci,* 2002 Jun;967:43-51

Phasic Insulin Release and Metabolic Regulation in Type 2 Diabetes. Stefano Del Prato et al. *Diabetes,* February 2002 vol. 51 no. suppl 1 S109-S116

Impaired Glucose Tolerance and Fasting Hyperglycaemia Have Different Characteristics. Davies MJ et al. *Diabet Med,* 2000 Jun;17(6):433-40

Impaired glucose tolerance and impaired fasting glycaemia: the current status on definition and intervention. Unwin N. et al. *Diabet Med,* 2002 Sep;19(9):708-23

Impaired early- but not late-phase insulin secretion in subjects with impaired fasting glucose. Mustafa Kanat et al. *Acta Diabetologica,* September 2011, Volume 48, Issue 3, pp 209-217

Beta Cell Dysfunction and Glucose Intolerance: Results from the San Antonio Metabolism (SAM) Study. Gastaldelli A et al. *Diabetologia,* 2004 Jan;47(1):31-9

Combined effects of single-nucleotide polymorphisms in GCK , GCKR , G6PC2 and MTNR1B on fasting plasma glucose and type 2 diabetes risk. E. Reiling et al. *Diabetologia,* September 2009, Volume 52, Issue 9, pp 1866-1870

Gender Differences in the Prevalence of Impaired Fasting Glycaemia and Impaired Glucose Tolerance in Mauritius. Does Sex Matter? Williams JW et al. *Diabet Med* 20 (11) 915 2003

ß-Cell Deficit and Increased ß-Cell Apoptosis in Humans with Type 2 Diabetes. Alexandra E. Butler et al. *Diabetes,* 52:102-110, 2003

Chapter Three: What Really Causes Diabetes?

Overweight and Obesity Statistics. NIH. http://www.niddk.nih.gov/health-information/health-statistics/Pages/overweight-obesity-statistics.aspx

CDC: Overweight and Obesity. http://www.cdc.gov/obesity/index.html

CDC: Diagnosed Diabetes. http://www.cdc.gov/diabetes/statistics/prev/national/figpersons.htm

National Diabetes Statistics Report. CDC.

   http//www.cdc.gov/diabetes/pubs/statsreport14/national-diabetes-report-web.pdf

Genome-wide association study in individuals of South Asian ancestry identifies six new type 2 diabetes susceptibility loci. Jaspal S. Kooner, et al. *Nature Genetics,* 2011

A variant near MTNR1B is associated with increased fasting plasma glucose levels and type 2 diabetes risk. Nabila Bouatia-Naji et al. *Nature Genetics,* 41, 89 - 94 (2008)

Beta cell glucose sensitivity is decreased by 39% in non-diabetic individuals carrying multiple diabetes-risk alleles compared with those with no risk alleles. L. Pascoe et al. *Diabetologia,* Volume 51, Number 11 / November, 2008

Clinical Risk Factors, DNA Variants, and the Development of Type 2 Diabetes. Valeriya Lyssenko et al. *N Engl J Med,* Volume 359:2220-2232, November 20, 2008, Number 21

The T allele of rs7903146 TCF7L2 is associated with impaired insuli-notropic action of incretin hormones, reduced 24 h profiles of plasma insulin and glucagon, and increased hepatic glucose production in young healthy men. K. Pilgaard et al. *Diabetologia,* Jul;52(7):1298-307

Glucose Tolerance in Adults after Prenatal Exposure to Famine. Ravelli AC, et al. *Lancet,* 1998 Jan 17;351(9097):173-7

Stable Patterns of Gene Expression Regulating Carbohydrate Metabolism Determined by Geographic Ancestry. Jonathan C. Schisler et al. *PLoS One,* 4(12): e8183

Adverse Metabolic Consequences in Humans of Prolonged Sleep Restriction Combined with Circadian Disruption. Orfeu M. Buxton et al. *Sci Transl Med,* 11 April 2012: Vol. 4, Issue 129, p. 129ra43

Subjects With Early-Onset Type 2 Diabetes Show Defective Activation of the Skeletal Muscle PGC-1α/Mitofusin-2 Regulatory Pathway in Response to Physical Activity. María Isabel Hernández-Alvarez, et al. *Diabetes Care,* March 2010 vol. 33 no. 3 645-651

Intrauterine Exposure to Environmental Pollutants and Body Mass Index during the First 3 Years of Life. Stijn L. Verhulst et al. *Environ Health Perspect,* January 2009, 117(1): 122-126

Prevalence of Obesity, Diabetes, and Obesity-Related Health Risk Factors, 2001. Ali H. Mokdad et al. *JAMA,* 2003;289:76-79

Chronic Exposure to the Herbicide, Atrazine, Causes Mitochondrial Dysfunction and Insulin Resistance. Soo Lim, et al. *PLoS ONE,* Published 13 Apr 2009

Arsenic Exposure and Prevalence of Type 2 Diabetes in US Adults. Ana Navas-Acien et al. *JAMA,* 2008;300(7):814-822

The Estrogenic Effect of Bisphenol-A Disrupts the Pancreatic β-Cell Function *In Vivo* and Induces Insulin Resistance. Alonso-Magdalena et al. *Environ Health Perspect,* 113(January):106-112

Diabetes in Relation to Serum Levels of Polychlorinated Biphenyls and Chlorinated Pesticides in Adult Native Americans. Neculai Codru et al. *Environ Health Perspect,* 2007 October; 115(10): 1442-1447

Prenatal Exposure to Perfluorooctanoate and Risk of Overweight at 20 Years of Age: A Prospective Cohort Study. Thorhallur I. Halldorsson et al. *Environ Health Perspect,* 2012 May;120(5):668-73

Perinatal Exposure to Bisphenol A at Reference Dose Predisposes Offspring to Metabolic Syndrome in Adult Rats on a High-Fat Diet. Jie Wei et al. *Endocrinology,* May 17, 2011

CBS News: New Study Finds High Levels of Phthalate Chemicals in Kid's Backpacks, Supplies. August 23, 2013. http://www.cbsnews.com/news/back-to-school-study-finds-high-levels-of-phthalate-chemicals-in-kids-backpacks-supplies/

Urinary Phthalates and Increased Insulin Resistance in Adolescents. Leonardo Trasande et al. *Pediatrics*, August 19, 2013, 2012-4022

Science Daily:Toxic Plastics: Bisphenol A Linked To Metabolic Syndrome In Human Tissue. September 5, 2008. http://www.sciencedaily.com/releases/2008/09/080904151629.htm

BPA-Free Plastic Containers May Be Just as Hazardous. Jenna Bilbrey. *Scientific American*, August 11, 2014

Simvastatin Improves Flow-Mediated Dilation but Reduces Adiponectin Levels and Insulin Sensitivity in Hypercholesterolemic Patient. Kwang Kon Koh et al., *Diabetes*, 31:776-782, 2008

Statin Use and Risk of Diabetes Mellitus in Postmenopausal Women in the Women's Health Initiative. Annie L. Culver et al. *Arch Intern Med*, 2012;172(2):144-152.

Risk of Incident Diabetes With Intensive-Dose Compared With Moderate-Dose Statin Therapy: A Meta-analysis. David Preiss et al. *JAMA*, 2011;305(24):2556-2564A

Meta-Analysis of 94,492 Patients With Hypertension Treated With Beta Blockers to Determine the Risk of New-Onset Diabetes Mellitus. Sripal Bangalore, et al. *Am J Cardiol*, 2007 Oct 15;100(8):1254-62

Antidepressant Use Associated with Increased Type 2 Diabetes Risk. Caroline Cassels. Medscape.com. Report on research paper presented at 2007 ADA convention. http://www.medscape.com/viewarticle/539078

Diabetes Mellitus in Long-term Survivors of Childhood Cancer: Increased Risk Associated With Radiation Therapy: A Report for the Childhood Cancer Survivor Study. Lillian R. Meacham et al. *Arch. Int. Med*, Vol. 169 No. 15, Aug 10/24, 2009

Downregulation of Diacylglycerol Kinase Delta Contributes to Hy-perglycemia-Induced Insulin Resistance. Alexander V. Chibalin et al. *Cell*, Volume 132, Issue 3, 375-386, 8 February 2008

Insulin Resistance in the First-Degree Relatives of Persons with Type 2 Diabetes. Straczkowski M et al. *Med Sci Monit*, 2003 May;9(5):CR186-90

Insulin Resistance in Children of Type 2 Parents who have Abnormal Mitochondria. Petersen KF et al. *N Engl J Med*, 2004 Feb 12; 350(7);639-41

Molecular Mechanisms of Insulin Resistance in Humans and Their Potential Links With Mitochondrial Dysfunction. Katsutaro Morino et al. *Diabetes*, 55:S9-S15, 2006

Chapter Four: Blood Sugar Level and Organ Damage

Increased Prevalence of Impaired Glucose Tolerance in Patients with Painful Sensory Neuropathy. Singleton, JR et al. *Diabetes Care*, 24 (8) 1448-1453 2001

The Spectrum of Neuropathy in Diabetes and Impaired Glucose Tolerance. J. Sumner et al. *Neurology*, 2003;60:108-111

Value of the Oral Glucose Tolerance Test in the Evaluation of Chronic Idiopathic Axonal Polyneuropathy. Charlene Hoffman-Snyder et al. *Arch Neurol*, 2006; 63:1075-1079

The Inflammatory Reflex. Kevin J. Tracey. *Nature*, 420, 853-859 (19 December 2002)

Inflammation markers and metabolic characteristics of subjects with one-hour plasma glucose levels. Gianluca Bardini et al. *Diabetes Care*, February 2010 33:411-413

Effect of an Intensive Glucose Management Protocol on the Mortality of Critically Ill Adult Patients. Krinsley, James. *Mayo Clinic Proc*, Jan 2004, p. 992-1000

ß-Cell Death and Mass in Syngeneically Transplanted Islets Exposed to Short- and Long-Term Hyperglycemia. Montserrat Biarnés et al. *Diabetes*, 51:66-72, 2002

Determinants of Glucose Toxicity and Its Reversibility in Pancreatic Islet Beta Cell Line, HIT-T15. Catherine E. Gleason et al. *Am J Physiol Endocrinol Metab*, 279: E997-E1002, 2000

ADA Scientific Sessions: Retinopathy Found in Prediabetes. Beckley, ET. *DOC News*, August 1, 2005. Volume 2 Number 8 p. 1

Association of A1C and Fasting Plasma Glucose Levels With Diabetic Retinopathy Prevalence in the U.S. Population: Implications for diabetes diagnostic thresholds Yiling J. Cheng et al. *Diabetes Care,* November 2009 vol. 32 no. 11 2027-2032.

Glycemic Thresholds for Diabetes-Specific Retinopathy: Implications for Diagnostic Criteria for Diabetes:The DETECT-2 Collaboration Writing group. Stephen Colagiuri et al. *Diabetes Care,* January 2011 vol. 34 no. 1 145-150

Hemoglobin A1c and Fasting Plasma Glucose Levels as Predictors of Retinopathy at 10 Years: The French DESIR Study. Massin P. et al. *Arch Ophthalmol,* 2011 Feb;129(2):188-195

Diabetic Retinopathy. Fong, DS et al. *Diabetes Care* October 2004 vol. 27 no. 10 2540-2553

Prospective Study of Hyperglycemia and Cancer Risk. Pär Stattin et al. *Diabetes Care,* 30:561-567, 2007

Fifty Percent of Patients with Coronary Artery Disease do Not Have Any of the Conventional Risk Factors. Futterman LG, Lemberg L. *Am J Crit Care,* 1998 May;7(3):240-4

Lipids, Risk Factors and Ischaemic Heart Disease. Castelli WP. *Atherosclerosis,* 1996 Jul;124 Suppl:S1-9

Post-challenge blood glucose concentration and stroke mortality rates in non-diabetic men in London: 38-year follow-up of the original Whitehall prospective cohort study. G. D. Batty et al. *Diabetologia,* Vol 51, Num, July, 2008

Association of Hemoglobin A1c with Cardiovascular Disease and Mortality in Adults: The European Prospective Investigation into Cancer in Norfolk Kay-Tee Khaw et al. *Ann Int Med,* Vol 141, no 6, 413-420

Cardiac Steatosis in Diabetes Mellitus: A 1H-Magnetic Resonance Spectroscopy Study. McGavock JM et al. *Circulation,* 2007 Sep 4;116(10):1170-5

Postmeal Glucose Peaks at Home Associate with Carotid Intima-Media Thickness in Type 2 Diabetes. Katherine Esposito et al. J *Clin Endocrinol Metab,* 2008 Apr;93(4):1345-50

Glycemic Control and Coronary Heart Disease Risk in Persons With and Without Diabetes. The Atherosclerosis Risk in Communities Study. Elizabeth Selvin et al. *Arch Intern Med.* 2005;165:1910-1916

Post-Challenge Glucose Predicts Coronary Atherosclerotic Progression inn Non-Diabetic, Post-Menopausal Women P. B. Mellen et al. *Diabetic Medicine,* 24 (10), 1156-1159

Glycation of LDL by Methylglyoxal Increases Arterial Atherogenicity: A Possible Contributor to Increased Risk of Cardiovascular Disease in Diabetes. Naila Rabbani et al. *Diabetes,* Published online before print May 26, 2011

Postprandial Blood Glucose Predicts Cardiovascular Events and All-Cause Mortality in Type 2 Diabetes in a 14-Year Follow-Up Lessons from the San Luigi Gonzaga Diabetes Study. Franco Cavalot et al. *Diabetes Care,* October 2011 vol. 34 no. 10 2237-2243

Intensive Blood Glucose Control and Vascular Outcomes in Patients with Type 2 Diabetes. The ADVANCE Collaborative Group. *N Engl J Med,* Volume 358:2560-2572, June 12, 2008, Number 24

Effects of Intensive Glucose Lowering in Type 2 Diabetes The Action to Control Cardiovascular Risk in Diabetes Study Group.[ACCORD] *N Engl J Med* Volume 358:2545-2559, June 12, 2008 Number 24

The ACCORD Study Group and ACCORD Eye Study Group. Effects of medical therapies on retinopathy progression in type 2 diabetes. *N Engl J Med* 2010 Jul 15; 363:233

Epidemiologic Relationships Between A1C and All-Cause Mortality During a Median 3.4-Year Follow-up of Glycemic Treatment in the ACCORD Trial. Matthew C. Riddle et al. *Diabetes Care* May 2010 vol. 33 no. 5 983-990

Poor Glycemic Control in Diabetes and the Risk of Incident Chronic Kidney Disease Even in the Absence of Albuminuria and Retinopathy: Atherosclerosis Risk in Communities (ARIC) Study. Lori D. Bash et al. *Arch Intern Med,* Vol. 168 No. 22, Dec 8/22, 2008

Short-term peaks in glucose promote renal fibrogenesis independ-ently of total glucose exposure.T. S. Polhill et al. *Am J Physiol Renal Physiol,* 287: F268-F273, 2004

Increased Incidence of Carpal Tunnel Syndrome up to 10 Years Before Diagnosis of Diabetes. Martin C. Gulliford et al. *Diabetes Care,* August 2006 vol. 29 no. 8 1929-1930

The prevalence of a diabetic condition and adhesive capsulitis of the shoulder. Tighe CB et al. *South Med J,* 2008 Jun;101(6):591-5

Thickness of the Supraspinatus and Biceps Tendons in Diabetic Patients. Mujde Akturk et al. *Diabetes Care,* February 2002 vol. 25 no. 2 40

Some Long-Term Sequelae of Poorly Controlled Diabetes that are Frequently Undiagnosed, Misdiagnosed or Mistreated. Richard K. Bernstein. http://www.diabetes-book.com/long-term-sequelae/

Short course prednisolone for adhesive capsulitis (frozen shoulder or stiff painful shoulder): a randomised, double blind, placebo controlled trial R Buchbinder et al. *Ann Rheum Dis* ,2004;63:1460-1469

Joslin's Diabetes Mellitus. C. Ronald Kahn et al. Lippincott Williams & Wilkins, 2005 p. 1064

Ligamentous Ossification of the Cervical Spine in the Late Middle-Aged Japanese Men: Its Relation to Body Mass Index and Glucose Metabolism. Shingyouchi, Yoshihiro et al. *Spine,* November 1, 1996 - Volume 21 - Issue 21

The influence of diabetes mellitus on lumbar intervertebral disk herniation. Sakellaridis *N. Surg Neurol,* 2006 Aug;66(2):152-4

Advanced glycation end products in degenerative nucleus pulposus with diabetes. Tsai, T. et al. *J Orthop Res,* 32: 238–244

Relationship Between GHb Concentration and Erythrocyte Survival Determined From Breath Carbon Monoxide Concentration. Mark A. Virtue, et al. *Diabetes Care,* April 2004 vol. 27 no. 4 931-935

A1C: Does One Size Fit All? Robert M. Cohen, *Diabetes Care,* October 2007 vol. 30 no. 10 2756-2758

Chapter Five: Must You Deteriorate?

Controlling the Diabetes: Just What Can You Achieve? Roy Taylor, M.D. http://www.medscape.com/viewarticle/460902_14

Diabetes Control and Complications Trial (DCCT) http://diabetes.niddk.nih.gov/dm/pubs/control/

UK Prospective Diabetes Study (UKPDS) http://www.dtu.ox.ac.uk/index.php?maindoc=/ukpds/

Long-Term Results of the Kumamoto Study on Optimal Diabetes Control in Type 2 Diabetic Patients. Motoaki Shichiri et al. *Diabetes Care,* Vol 23 Sup 2, 2000

Effects of Duration of Type 2 Diabetes Mellitus on Insulin Secretion. Farhad Zangeneh, Puneet S. Arora et al. *Endocr Pract,* 2006;12:388-393

Chapter Six: How to Lower Blood Sugar

FDA: Shasta Technologies GenStrip Blood Glucose Test Strips May Report False Results: FDA Safety Communication.

FDA: Class 2 Device Recall UniStrip1

Dr. Bernstein's Diabetes Solution: The Complete Guide to Achieving Normal Blood Sugars, 3rd Ed. Richard K. Bernstein. Little Brown, New York, 2007, ISBN 978-0316167161. p. 259

Protein Power. Michael R. Eades and Mary Dan Eades, Bantam Books, 199.

The earliest references to The 5% Club is found in this alt.support.diabetes posting: http://groups.google.com/group/alt.support.diabetes/browse_frm/thread/40c55ce608d68b4e/

AACE American Association of Clinical Endocrinologists Medical Guidelines for Developing a Diabetes Mellitus Comprehensive Care Plan - 2011. https://www.aace.com/files/dm-guidelines-ccp.pdf

Evolution in the American Diabetes Association Standards of Care. John B. Buse, *Clinical Diabetes,* 21:24-26, 2003

Washington Post. For Decades the Government Steered Millions Away from Whole Milk. Was that Wrong? Oct. 6, 2015

Reversal of type 2 diabetes: normalisation of beta cell function in association with decreased pancreas and liver triacylglycerol. Lim EL, et al. *Diabetologia, 2011 Oct;54(10):2506-14*

Restoring normoglycaemia by use of a very low calorie diet in long- and short-duration Type 2 diabetes. Steven S et al. *Diabet Med,* 2015 Sep;32(9):1149-55

Activists Facts: Physicians Committee for Responsible Medicine. https://www.activistfacts.com/organizations/23-physicians-committee-for-responsible-medicine/

Can Diabetes Be Surgically Cured? Long-Term Metabolic Effects of Bariatric Surgery in Obese Patients with Type 2 Diabetes Mellitus. Brethauer, Stacy A et al. *Ann Surg*, October 2013 - Volume 258 - Issue 4 - p 628–637

Chapter Seven: Making the Diet Work

Comparison of the Atkins, Ornish, Weight Watchers, and Zone Diets for Weight Loss and Heart Disease Risk Reduction. A Randomized Trial. Michael L. Dansinger et al. *JAMA*, 2005;293:43-53

Comparison of the Atkins, Zone, Ornish, and LEARN Diets for Change in Weight and Related Risk Factors Among Overweight Premenopausal Women. Christopher D. Gardner et al. *JAMA*, 2007;297:969-977

Effect of a High-Protein, Low-Carbohydrate Diet on Blood Glucose Control in People with Type 2 Diabetes. Mary C. Gannon et al. *Diabetes*, 53:2375-2382, 2004

Effect of a Low-Carbohydrate Diet on Appetite, Blood Glucose Levels, and Insulin Resistance in Obese Patients with Type 2 Diabetes. Guenther Boden et al. *Ann Intern Med*, 2005 Mar 15;142(6):403-11

The Effects of Low-Carbohydrate Versus Conventional Weight Loss Diets in Severely Obese Adults: One-Year Follow-up of a Randomized Trial. Stern L et al. *Ann Intern Med*, 2004 May 18; 140(10):778-85

Diet 101: The Truth About Low Carb Diets, Jenny Ruhl, Technion Books, Turners Falls, 2012 ISBN 978-0-9647116-5-5. (pp. 61-69 discuss the research on long term low carb diet failure. pp 88-89 discusses MSG research.)

Fructose, Weight Gain, and the Insulin Resistance Syndrome. Sharon S. Elliott et al. *Am J Clin Nutr*, Vol 76 No. 5 911-922, 2002

Experimental Studies on the Role of Fructose in the Development of Diabetic Complications. Sakai M, Oimomi M et al. *J Med Sci,*, Dec 2002, 48(5-6) p125-36

Phosphate Additives Promote Hardening of the Arteries. http://diabetesupdate.blogspot.com/2013/06/phosphate-additives-promote-hardening.html (contains links to research cited.)

Atkins Under Attack. Mary Carmichael , *Newsweek*, 2/22/04 AT 7:00 PM

Perennial Foes Meet Again in a Battle of the Snack Bar. Joe Sharkey. *New York Times*, Nov. 23, 2004

Intake of saturated and trans unsaturated fatty acids and risk of all cause mortality, cardiovascular disease, and type 2 diabetes: systematic review and meta-analysis of observational studies, DeSouza, RJ et al. *BMJ*, 2015; 351(Published 12 August 2015)

Can Diabetes Be Surgically Cured? Long-Term Metabolic Effects of Bariatric Surgery in Obese Patients with Type 2 Diabetes Mellitus. Brethauer, Stacy A. et al. *Ann Surg*, October 2013 - Volume 258 - Issue 4 - p 628–637

Mortality Rate Associated with Bariatric Surgery Reaches New Lows, Life Expectancy Reaches New Highs. http://connect.asmbs.org/february-2015-surgery-mortality.html

New Procedure Estimates for Bariatric Surgery: What the Statistics Reveal. http://connect.asmbs.org/may-2014-bariatric-surgery-growth.html

Chapter Eight: Generic Diabetes Drugs

The FDA mandated "**Prescribing Information**" for all drugs can be found in the *Physicians Desk Reference* (PDR) or search for it on the web. Your pharmacist can also give you a copy

Metformin and Insulin Suppress Hepatic Gluconeogenesis through Phosphorylation of CREB Binding Protein. Ling He et al, *Cell*, Volume 137, Issue 4, 635-646, 15 May 2009

Metformin Increases AMP-Activated Protein Kinase Activity in Skeletal Muscle of Subjects with Type 2 Diabetes. Nicolas Musi et al. *Diabetes*, 51: 2074-2081

AMP-Activated Protein Kinase Conducts the Ischemic Stress Response Orchestra. Lawrence H. Young. *Circulation*, 2008;117:832-840

Enhanced secretion of glucagon-like peptide 1 by biguanide compounds. Yasuda N et al. *Biochem Biophys Res Commun*, 2002 Nov 15;298(5):779-84

New Users of Metformin Are at Low Risk of Incident Cancer: A cohort study among people with type 2 diabetes. Gillian Libby et al. *Diabetes Care,* September 2009 vol. 32 no. 9 1620-1625.

Science Daily: Diabetes Drug Kills Cancer Stem Cells in Combination Treatment in Mice. http://www.sciencedaily.com/releases/2009/09/090914110530.htm

Metformin Associated With Lower Cancer Mortality in Type 2 Diabetes: ZODIAC-16 Gijs W.D. Landman et al. *Diabetes Care,* February 2010 vol. 33 no. 2 322-326

Metformin Treatment Exerts Antiinvasive and Antimetastatic Effects in Human Endometrial Carcinoma Cells. *J. Clin. Endo &Metab*, 2010; 96 (3): 808

Diabetes, Metformin, and Breast Cancer in Postmenopausal Women. Rowan T. Chlebowski et al. *J Clin Oncol,* 2012 Aug 10;30(23):2844-52

Metformin Does Not Affect Cancer Risk: A Cohort Study in the U.K. Clinical Practice Research Datalink Analyzed Like an Intention-to-Treat Trial. Konstantinos K. Tsilidis et al. *Diabetes Care,* 2014 Sep;37(9):2522-32

Long-term Effects of Metformin on Metabolism and Microvascular and Macrovascular Disease in Patients With Type 2 Diabetes Mellitus. Kooy et all. *Arch Int Med,* 169 (6), 616-625

Can people with type 2 diabetes live longer than those without? A comparison of mortality in people initiated with metformin or sulphonylurea monotherapy and matched, non-diabetic controls. A. Bannister, et al. *Diabetes ObesMetab,* Vol 16, Issue 11, pps 1165–1173, Nov 2014

Secondary Failure of Metformin Monotherapy in Clinical Practice. Jonathan B. Brown. *Diabetes Care*, March 2010 vol. 33 no. 3 501-506

Incidence of Lactic Acidosis in Metformin Users. Stang M et al. *Diabetes Care,* Jun 1999, 22(6) p925-7

Risk of Fatal and Nonfatal Lactic Acidosis with Metformin Use in Type 2 Diabetes Mellitus: Systematic Review and Meta-Analysis. Salpeter SR et al. *Arch Intern Med,* 2003 Nov 24;163(21):2594-602.

Effects of Short-Term Treatment with Metformin on Serum Concentrations of Homocysteine, Folate and Vitamin B12 in Type 2 Diabetes Mellitus: A Randomized, Placebo-Controlled Trial. Wulffele MG et al. *J Intern Med,* 2003 Nov;254(5):455-63.

Increased Risk of Cognitive Impairment in Patients With Diabetes Is Associated With Metformin. Eileen M. Moore, et al., *Diabetes Care,* October 2013 vol. 36 no. 10 2981-2987

Metformin Cuts Dementia Risk in Type 2 Diabetes.
   http://www.medscape.com/viewarticle/807886 (July 16, 2013)

Incidence of dementia is increased in type 2 diabetes and reduced by the use of sulfonylureas and metformin. Hsu CC, et al. *J Alzheimers Dis,* 2011;24(3):485-93.

Metformin in the diabetic brain: friend or foe? Paula I. Moreira. *Ann Transl Med,* 2014 Jun; 2(6): 54.

Effects of the Alpha-Glucosidase Inhibitor Acarbose on the Development of Long-Term Complications in Diabetic Animals: Pathophysioloical and Therapeutic Implications. Creutzfeldt W. *Diabetes Metab Res,* rev. 1999 15(4):289-96

STOP-NIDDM Trial Research Group. Acarbose for Prevention of Type 2 Diabetes Mellitus: the STOP-NIDDM Randomised Trial. Chiasson JL et al. *Lancet,* 2002 Jun 15;359 (9323):2072-7

Dose-Response Relation Between Sulfonylurea Drugs and Mortality in Type 2 Diabetes Mellitus: A Population-Based Cohort Study. Scot H. Simpson, et al. *CMAJ,* January 17, 2006; 174

Risk of coronary artery disease associated with initial sulphonylurea treatment of patients with type 2 diabetes: A matched case-control study Shaukat M. Sadikot et al. *Diabetes Res Clil Pract,* Volume 82, Issue 3, December 2008, Pages 391-395

Metformin, Sulfonylureas, or Other Antidiabetes Drugs and the Risk of Lactic Acidosis or Hypoglycemia: A nested case-control analysis. Michael Bodmer et. at. *Diabetes Care,* 31:2086-2091, 2008

Chronic Antidiabetic Sulfonylureas In Vivo: Reversible Effects on Mouse Pancreatic ß-Cells. Remedi MS et al. *PLoS Med,* 5(10): e206

Effects of antidiabetic drugs on dipeptidyl peptidase IV activity: nateglinide is an inhibitor *of DPP IV and augments the antidiabetic activity of glucagon-like peptide-1. Duffy NA et al. Eur J Pharmacol,* 2007 Jul 30;568(1-3):278-86

Chronic Antidiabetic Sulfonylureas In Vivo: Reversible Effects on Mouse Pancreatic ß-Cells. Remedi MS et al. *PLoS Med,* 5(10): e206

Scientist Says Executive of Avandia Firm Tried to Bully. Study by Researcher Tied Drug to Heart Ills. Diedtra Henderson, *Boston Globe,* June 7, 2007

Thiazolidinediones and Heart Failure: A Teleo-Analysis. Sonal Singh et al. *Diabetes Care,* August 2007 vol. 30 no. 8 2148-2153

Effects of Pioglitazone Versus Diet and Exercise on Metabolic Health and Fat Distribution in Upper Body Obesity. Samyah Shadid, MD and Michael D. Jensen, MD. *Diabetes Care,* 26:3148-3152, 2003

Thiazolidinedione-Associated Congestive Heart Failure and Pulmonary Edema. Kermani A, Garg A. *Mayo Clin Proc,* 2003 Sep;78(9):1088-91

Glitazone Use May Be Associated with Macular Edema in Diabetics. Karla Harby. http://www.medscape.com/viewarticle/464732

Hepatotoxicity of the Thiazolidinediones. Tolman KG, Chandramouli. *J. Clin Liver Dis,* May 2003, 7(2) p369-79

Long-term use of thiazolidinediones and fractures in type 2 diabetes: a meta-analysis. Yoon K. Loke et al. *CMAJ, 2009 Jan 6;180(1):32-9*

Thiazolidinedione Use and the Longitudinal Risk of Fractures in Patients with Type 2 Diabetes. Mellitus Zeina A. Habib et al. *J Clin Endo & Metab,* Vol. 95, No. 2 592-600

FDA reviewing preliminary safety information on Actos

FDA Drug Safety Communication: Update to ongoing safety review of Actos (pioglitazone) and increased risk of bladder cancer

FDA News Release: FDA requires removal of certain restrictions on the diabetes drug Avandia

FDA reverses course on Avandia warning, lifts safety restrictions. CBS News 11/25/13

Peroxisome Proliferator-activated Receptor gamma Controls Ingestive Behavior, AgRP, and NPY mRNA in the Arcuate Hypothalamus. Garretson JT et al. *Neuroscience,* 2015; 35(11): 4571-81

Chapter Nine: Patented Diabetes Drugs

BYETTA® Study Showed Sustained Blood Glucose Control Over Three Years in People with Type 2 Diabetes. Lilly Amylin PR Newswire press release. June 25, 2007

Merck 2014 Annual Report. http://www.merck.com/investors/financials/annual-reports/home.html

Top 50 Pharmaceutical Products by Global Sales. http://www.pmlive.com/top_pharma_list/Top_50_pharmaceutical_products_by_global_s ales

Safety and tolerability of sitagliptin in clinical studies: a pooled analysis of data from 10,246 patients with type 2 diabetes. Debora Williams-Herman et al. [at Merck] *BMC Endocrine Disorders,* 2010, 10:7

FDA Drug Safety Communication: FDA warns that DPP-4 inhibitors for type 2 diabetes may cause severe joint pain

CD26 [DPP-4] Is Negatively Associated with Inflammation in Human and Experimental Arthritis. Nathalie Busso et al. *Am J Pathol,* 2005;166:433-442

Studies of DPP-4 gene function: http://www.ihop-net.org/UniPub/iHOP/bng/87784.html

A Role for Dipeptidyl Peptidase IV in Suppressing the Malignant Phenotype of Melanocytic Cells. Umadevi V. Wesleya et al. *J Exp Med,* Volume 190, Number 3, August 2, 1999 311-322

CD26/dipeptidyl peptidase IV regulates prostate cancer metastasis by degrading SDF-1/CXCL12. Sun YX et al, *Clin Exp Metastasis,* 2008;25(7):765-76

Dipeptidyl Peptidase IV (DPPIV) Inhibits Cellular Invasion of Melanoma Cells. Pethiyagoda CL et al. *Clin Exp Metastasis,* 2001, 18:391-400

Prolonged Survival and Decreased Invasive Activity Attributable to Dipeptidyl Peptidase IV Overexpression in Ovarian Carcinoma. Hiroaki Kajiyama et al. *Cancer Research,* 62, 2753-2757, May 15, 2002

A Critical Analysis of the Clinical Use of Incretin-Based Therapies:Are the GLP-1 therapies safe? Peter C. Butler, et al. *Diabetes Care,* 2013 Jul; 36(7): 2118–2125

Beneficial Endocrine but Adverse Exocrine Effects of Sitagliptin in the Human Islet Amyloid Polypeptide Transgenic Rat Model of Type 2 Diabetes. Interactions With Metformin, Aleksey V. Matveyenko1, et al. *Diabetes,* July 2009 vol. 58 no. 7 1604-1615

Acute Pancreatitis in Type 2 Diabetes Treated With Exenatide or Sitagliptin: A retrospective observational pharmacy claims analysis. Rajesh Garg et al. Diabetes Care, Nov 2010 vol. 33 no. 11 2349-2354

Glucagon like peptide 1-based therapies and risk of hospitalization for acute pancreatitis in type 2 diabetes mellitus: a population-based matched case-control study. Singh S, et al. *JAMA Intern Med* 2013 Feb 25:1-6

FDA: Information for Healthcare Professionals - Acute pancreatitis and sitaglipitn.

Marked Expansion of Exocrine and Endocrine Pancreas with Incretin Therapy in Humans with increased Exocrine Pancreas Dysplasia and the potential for Glucagon-producing Neuroendocrine Tumors. Butler, AE, et al. *Diabetes,* July 2013 vol. 62 no. 7 2595-2604

Pancreatitis, Pancreatic, and Thyroid Cancer With Glucagon-Like Peptide-1–Based Therapies. Michael Elashoff et al. *Gastroenterology,* 2011;141:150–156

Effect of Sitagliptin on Cardiovascular Outcomes in Type 2 Diabetes. Jennifer B. Green, et al. *N Engl J Med* 2015; 373:232-242

Invokana FDA Approved Prescribing Information

Farxiga FDA Approved Prescribing Information

Jardiance FDA Approved Prescribing Information

FDA Safety Information for Byetta

FDA Drug Safety Communication: FDA warns that SGLT2 inhibitors for diabetes may result in a serious condition of too much acid in the blood

FDA Drug Safety Communication. Invokamet (canagliflozin): New Information on Bone Fracture Risk and Decreased Bone Mineral Density

Lilly Press Release. Jardiance® (empagliflozin) is the only diabetes medication to show a significant reduction in both cardiovascular risk and cardiovascular death in a dedicated outcome trial

Empagliflozin, Cardiovascular Outcomes, and Mortality in Type 2 Diabetes. Bernard Zinman et al. *N Engl J Med,* Published online September 17, 2015 with Supplementary Appendix

Chapter Ten: Insulin

Randomized Trial on the Influence of the Length of Two Insulin Pen Needles on Glycemic Control and Patient Preference in Obese Patients with Diabetes. Gillian Kreugel, et al. *Diabetes Technol Ther,* July 2011, 13(7): 737-741

Think Like a Pancreas: A Practical Guide to Managing Diabetes with Insulin. 2nd Ed. Gary Scheiner. Marlowe, 2012

Dr. Bernstein's Diabetes Solution, op. cit.

Using Insulin, Everything You Need for Success With Insulin. John Walsh et al. Torrey Pines Press. 2003

FDA Approved Prescribing Information for all insulins discussed.

Chapter Eleven: Supplements and Healing Foods

DNA barcoding detects contamination and substitution in North American herbal products. Steven G Newmaster, et al. *BMC Med,* 2013, 11:222

Major Retailers Ordered to Stop Selling 'Adulterated' and 'Mislabeled' Supplements. News Desk. *Food Safety News.* February 3, 2015

Insulin Potentiating Factor and Chromium Content of Selected Foods and Spices. Khan A, Bryden et al. *Biol Trace Elem Res,* 1990 Mar;24(3):183-8

Cinnamon supplementation does not improve glycemic control in postmenopausal type 2 diabetes patients. Vanschoonbeek K et al., *J Nutr,* 2006 Apr;136(4):977-80

The Effect of Cinnamon on Glucose Control and Lipid Parameters William L Baker, et al. *Diabetes Care,* October 1, 2007

Elevated Intakes of Supplemental Chromium Improve Glucose and Insulin Variables in Individuals with Type 2 Diabetes. RA Anderson et al. *Diabetes,* Vol 46, Issue 11 1786-1791

Chromium, Glucose Intolerance and Diabetes. Richard A. Anderson, *J Am Coll Nutr,* Vol. 17, No. 6, 548-555 (1998)

Glucose and Insulin Responses to Dietary Chromium Supplements: A Meta-Analysis. Althuis et al. *Am J Clin Nutr,* 2002 Jul;76(1):148-55

Chromium (III) Tris (Picolinate) is Mutagenic at the Hypoxanthine (Guanine) Phosphoribosyltransferase Locus in Chinese Hamster Ovary Cells. Stearns DM et al. *Mutat Res,* Jan 15 2002, 513(1-2) p135-42

MRC/BHF Heart Protection Study of Antioxidant Vitamin Supplementation in 20,536 High-Risk Individuals: A Randomised Placebo-Controlled Trial. Heart Protection Study Collaborative Group. *Lancet,* Jul 6 2002, 360(9326) p23-33

Vitamin C and Hyperglycemia in the European Prospective Investigation into Cancer—Norfolk (EPIC-Norfolk) study: a Population-based Study. Sargeant LA et al. *Diabetes Care,* Jun 2000, 23(6) p726-32

Occupational Social Class, Educational Level and Area Deprivation Independently Predict Plasma Ascorbic Acid Concentration: A Cross-Sectional Population Based Study in the Norfolk Cohort of the European Prospective Investigation Into Cancer (EPIC-Norfolk). Shohaimi S et al. *Eur J Clin Nutr,* Mar 31 2004

Double-Blind, Randomised Study of the Effect of Combined Treatment With Vitamin C And E on Albuminuria in Type 2 Diabetic Patients. Gaede P, Poulsen et al. *Diabet Med,* Sep 2001, 18(9) p756-60

Mortality in Randomized Trials Of Antioxidant Supplements for Primary and Secondary Prevention: Systematic Review and Meta-Analysis. Bjelakovic G, Nikolova D et al. *JAMA,* 2007 Feb 28;297(8):842-57

Antioxidants May Make Cancer Worse: New animal studies explain why supposedly healthy supplements like beta-carotene could exacerbate a dread disease. Melinda Wenner Moyer. *Scientific American.* October 7, 2015

Treatment of type 2 diabetes and dyslipidemia with the natural plant alkaloid berberine. Zhang Y. *J Clin Endocrinol Metab,* 2008 Jul;93(7):2559-65.

WebMD: Berberine/Interactions. http://www.webmd.com/vitamins-supplements/ingredientmono-1126-berberine.aspx?activeingredientid=1126&activeingredientname=berberine

A Miracle Diabetes Cure. Gretchen Becker.

http://www.healthcentral.com/diabetes/c/5068/19892/miracle-cure/

Dr. Bernstein's Diabetes Solution, op. cit. p. 246

Oral Administration of RAC-Alpha-Lipoic Acid Modulates Insulin Sensitivity in Patients with Type-2 Diabetes Mellitus: A Placebo-Controlled Pilot Trial. Jacob S, Ruus P et al. *Free Radic Biol Med,* Aug 1999, 27(3-4) p309-14

Oral Treatment With Alpha-Lipoic Acid Improves Symptomatic Diabetic Polyneuropathy. The SYDNEY Trial. Dan Ziegler et al. *Diabetes Care,* 29:2365-2370, 2006

Alpha-Lipoic Acid: A Multifunctional Antioxidant that Improves Insulin Sensitivity in Patients with Type 2 Diabetes. Evans JL, Goldfine ID. *Diabetes Technol Ther,* Autumn 2000, 2(3) p401-13

Magnesium Intake and Risk of Type 2 Diabetes in Men And Women. Ruy Lopez-Ridaura et al. *Diabetes Care,* 27:134-140, 2003

Dietary Magnesium Intake in Relation to Plasma Insulin Levels and Risk of Type 2 Diabetes in Women. Lopez-Ridaura R et al. *Diabetes Care,* 27:59-65, 2003

The Whole Soy Story: The Dark Side of America's Favorite Health Food. Kaayla T. Daniel, Ph.D. NewTrends Publishing, Inc, 2005

Use of Soy Protein Supplement and Resultant Need for Increased Dose of Levothyroxine. Bell DS et al. *Endocr Pract,* 2001 May-Jun;7(3):193-4

The Role of Vitamin D and Calcium in Type 2 Diabetes. A Systematic Review and Meta-Analysis. Anastassios G. Pittas et al. *J Clin Endo & Metab,* Vol. 92, No. 6 2017-2029

Oral Administration of RAC-Alpha-Lipoic Acid Modulates Insulin Sensitivity in Patients with Type-2 Diabetes Mellitus: A Placebo-Controlled Pilot Trial. Jacob S et al. *Free Radic Biol Med,* Aug 1999, 27(3-4) p309-14

Alpha-Lipoic Acid: A Multifunctional Antioxidant that Improves Insulin Sensitivity in Patients with Type 2 Diabetes. Evans JL, et al. *Diabetes Technol Ther,* Autumn 2000, 2(3) p401-13

Benfotiamine Prevents Macro- and Microvascular Endothelial Dysfunction and Oxidative Stress Following a Meal Rich in Advanced Glycation End Products in Individuals With Type 2 Diabetes. Alin Stirban, et al. *Diabetes Care,* 29:2064-2071, 2006

Benfotiamine Blocks Three Major Pathways of Hyperglycemic Damage and Prevents Experimental Diabetic Retinopathy. Hans-Peter Hammes et al. *Nat Med,* 9, 294-299 (2003)

Benfotiamine in the Treatment of Diabetic Polyneuropathy: A Three-Week Randomized, Controlled Pilot Study (BEDIP Study). Haupt E, Ledermann et al. *Int J Clin Pharmacol Ther,* 2005 Feb;43(2):71-7

The Effects of Long-Term Oral Benfotiamine Supplementation on Peripheral Nerve Function and Inflammatory Markers in Patients With Type 1 Diabetes: A 24-month, double-blind, randomized, placebo-controlled trial. David A. Fraser et al. *Diabetes Care,* May 2012 vol. 35 no. 5 1095-1097

Comment from Dan Ziegler et al. on: Fraser et al. The Effects of Long-Term Oral Benfotiamine Supplementation on Peripheral Nerve Function and Inflammatory Markers in Patients With Type 1 Diabetes. *Diabetes Care,* November 2012 vol. 35 no. 11 e79 (Pointing out flaws in the cited study design.)

Serum 25-Hydroxyvitamin D Concentration and Subsequent Risk of Type 2 Diabetes. Catharina Mattila et al. *Diabetes Care,* 30:2569-2570, 2007

Glucose tolerance and vitamin D: Effects of treating vitamin D deficiency. Kamilia Tai. *Nutrition,* Volume 24, Issue 10, Pages 950-956 (October 2008)

The effect of different doses of vitamin D3 on markers of vascular health in patients with type 2 diabetes: a randomised controlled trial. M. D. Witham et al. *Diabetologia,* Volume 53, Number 10, 2112-2119

Vitamin D Deficiency and Risk of Cardiovascular Disease. Thomas J. Wang et al. *Circulation,* 2008;117:503-511.

Serum Vitamin D Concentration Does Not Predict Insulin Action or Secretion in European Subjects With the Metabolic Syndrome. Hanne L. Gulseth et al. *Diabetes Care,* April 2010 vol. 33 no. 4 923-925

Association of Oral Calcitriol w*ith Improved Survival in Nondialyzed CKD. Abigail B. Shoben et al.* J Am Soc Nephrol, 2008 Aug;19(8):1613-9

Got Calcium? Welcome to the Calcium-Alkali Syndrome. Ami M. Patel and Stanley Goldfarb. *J Am Soc Nephro;* 21: 1440-1443, 2010

Vanadium & Diabetes, Benefit or Harm? John Walsh. http://www.diabetesnet.com/vanadium-diabetes

Coenzyme Q10 improves blood pressure and glycaemic control: a controlled trial in subjects with type 2 diabetes. Hodgson JM, *Eur J Clin Nutr,* 2002 Nov;56(11):1137-42

Statins May Actually Cause Diabetes.

http://phlauntdiabetesupdates.blogspot.com/2012/01/statins-may-actually-cause-diabetes.html

Statin Use and Risk of Diabetes Mellitus in Postmenopausal Women in the Women's Health Initiative. Annie L. Culver et al. *Arch Intern Med,* 2012;172(2):144-152

Risk of Incident Diabetes With Intensive-Dose Compared With Moderate-Dose Statin Therapy: A Meta-analysis David Preiss et al. *JAMA,* 2011;305(24):2556-2564.

Effect of hydrosoluble coenzyme Q10 on blood pressures and insulin resistance in hypertensive patients with coronary artery disease. Singh RB et al: *J Hum Hypertens,* (1999) 13, 203-208

Effects of High vs Low Glycemic Index of Dietary Carbohydrate on Cardiovascular Disease Risk Factors and Insulin Sensitivity. The OmniCarb Randomized Clinical Trial, Frank M. Sacks, et al. *JAMA,* 2014;312(23):2531-2541

Chapter Twelve: Exercise

Knee Replacement and Revision Surgeries on the Rise. Linda Rath. Arthritis Foundation. http://www.arthritis.org/living-with-arthritis/treatments/joint-surgery/types/knee/knee-replacement-younger-patients.php

Effects of Exercise on Glycemic Control and Body Mass in Type 2 Diabetes Mellitus: A Meta-analysis of Controlled Clinical Trials. Boulé N G, et al. *JAMA*, 2001;286:1218-1227

Intensity and Amount of Physical Activity in Relation to Insulin Sensitivity: The Insulin Resistance Atherosclerosis Study. Elizabeth J. Mayer-Davis et al. *JAMA*, 1998;279:669-674.

What are the risks of sitting too much ?James A. Levine, Mayo Clinic http://www.mayoclinic.org/healthy-lifestyle/adult-health/expert-answers/sitting/faq-20058005

Target Heart Rate. American Heart Association.
http://www.americanheart.org/presenter.jhtml?identifier=4736

Some Long-Term Sequelae of Poorly Controlled Diabetes that are Frequently Undiagnosed, Misdiagnosed or Mistreated. Richard K. Bernstein. http://www.diabetes-book.com/articles/poorly_controlled_diabetes.shtml

Carpal Tunnel May Predict Diabetes (WebMD):
http://diabetes.webmd.com/news/20060822/carpal-tunnel-predict-diabetes

Thickness of the Supraspinatus and Biceps Tendons in Diabetic Patients. Mujde Akturk et al. *Diabetes Care*, 25:408, 2002

Dr. Bernstein's Diabetes Solution, op. cit. 214-222

Using Pedometers to Increase Physical Activity and Improve Health: A Systematic Review. Dena M. Bravata, MD et al. *JAMA*, 2007;298(19):2296-2304

Standing-based office work shows encouraging signs of attenuating post-prandial glycaemic excursion. John P Buckley, et al. *Occup Environ Med*, published online December 2, 2013

Keeping it Off: Winning at Weight Loss. Robert H. Olson and Susan C. Colvin. Gilliland, 1989

Normal weight men and women overestimate exercise energy expenditure. Willbond SM et al. *J Sports Med Phys Fitness*, (2010) 50(4):377-84

Chapter Thirteen: Is it Really Type 2

University of Chicago: Types of MODY. http://monogenicdiabetes.uchicago.edu/what-is-monogenic-diabetes/mody-maturity-onset-diabetes-of-the-young/types-of-mody/

Athena Diagnostics: Testing and Diagnosis. http://www.modyawareness.com/healthcare-professionals/testing-diagnosis.php

Latent Autoimmune Diabetes Of Adulthood: Unique Features that Distinguish It From Types 1 and 2. Fadi Nabhan et al. *Postgraduate Medicine*, Vol 117, No 3, Mar 2005

Genetic Similarities Between LADA, Type 1 and Type 2 Diabetes. Camilla Cervin et al. *Diabetes*, 2008 May;57(5):1433-7

Common variants in the TCF7L2 gene help to differentiate autoimmune from non-autoimmune diabetes in young (15–34 years) but not in middle-aged (40–59 years) diabetic patients. E. Bakhtadze et al. *Diabetologia*, 2008 Dec;51(12):2224-32

Identification of MODY: The Implications for Holly. Jo Dalton, Maggie Shepherd. *J Diabetes Nurs*, Jan, 2004

Insights into the Beta-cell from patients with monogenic diabetes. Andrew Hattersley. EASD lecture, Sept 15, 2015

Determinants of the Development of Diabetes (Maturity-Onset Diabetes of the Young- in Carriers of HNF-1{alpha} Mutations. Evidence for Parent-of-Origin Effect. Tomasz Klupa, et al. *Diabetes Care*, 25:2292-2301, 2002

Altered Insulin Secretory Responses to Glucose In Diabetic and Nondiabetic Subjects with Mutations in the Diabetes Susceptibility Gene MODY3 on Chromosome 12MM. Byrne et al. *Diabetes* Vol 45, Issue 11 1503-1510

Assessment of Insulin Sensitivity in Glucokinase-Deficient Subjects. Clement K et al. *Diabetes Care*, 25:2292-2301, 2002

Prevalence of vascular complications among patients with glucokinase mutations and prolonged, mild hyperglycemia. Steele AM et al. *JAMA,* 2014 Jan 15;311(3):279-86

A low renal threshold for glucose in diabetic patients with a mutation in the hepatocyte nuclear factor-1alpha (HNF-1alpha) gene. Menzel R et al. *Diabet Med,* 1998 Oct;15(10):816-20.

Genes and Diabetes: Molecular and Clinical Characterization of Mutations in Transcription Factors. Timothy M. Frayling et al. *Diabetes,* Vol. 50, Sup 1, Feb 2001

Genetic Types of Diabetes Including MODY (UK - Exeter Research & Testing) http://www.projects.ex.ac.uk/diabetesgenes/

Diagnosis and Management of Maturity-Onset Diabetes of the Young. Timsit, Jose et al. *Treat in Endo* 4(1):9-18, 2005 (Contains finding that parents carrying gene may not have been diagnosed)

Chapter Fourteen: Working with Doctors and Hospitals

American Association of Clinical Endocrinologists: Most Recent AACE Guidelines.http://www.aace.com/pub/guidelines/

Diabetes in Control. http://diabetesincontrol.com

Dr. Bernstein's Diabetes Solution. op cit. Appendix B p. 462. Sample doctor letter

Medical research is surprisingly silent on the topic of the competence of medical practitioners. This chapter draws mostly on thousands of anecdotal reports posted by people with diabetes who have achieved excellent control.

Appendix B: What Can You Eat?

Recipes for Indispensable Low Carb Treats. http://www.phlaunt.com/diabetes/43067291.php

The Low-Carb Comfort Food Cookbook. Michael R. Eades et al.Wiley, 2002. Magic Rolls are on P. 22.

500 Low-Carb Recipes: 500 Recipes from Snacks to Dessert, That the Whole Family Will Love. Dana Carpender. Fair Winds Press, 2002.

Acknowledgements

This book grew out of years of daily interaction with hundreds of people active in the online diabetes community, each one of whom has contributed something valuable. My thanks to all!

I learned a great deal from the many people who posted informative messages on the alt.support.diabetes newsgroup between 1998 and 2005. I also owe a huge debt to Jennifer (last name unknown), whose "good advice" was the basis for the simple but powerful "Test, test, test" strategy taught in this book.

Special thanks are also due to Alan Shanley., Alice Faber, Annette, Chakolate, Chris Malcolm, GysdeJongh, Jefferson a.k.a. Frank Roy, Julie Bove, Loretta, Mack, Nicky, Old Al, Ottercritter, Ozgirl, Priscilla H Ballou, Ratty, Susan, W. Baker, Ted Rosenberg, and Wes Groleau.

RIP Quentin Grady, your sharp insights and wit are greatly missed.

When preparing the material for this new edition I also received valuable feedback from the many people who have posted comments on my blog and short-lived FaceBook page.

I have also benefited from the steady stream of readers who have emailed me with questions that weren't answered on the web site or in the first edition of this book. They helped me further refine both. In this new edition I hope I have covered the most common questions they contacted me about that weren't covered in the first edition.

I am fortunate to have Gretchen Becker as a friend. She keeps me grounded when I indulge in too much speculation and comes up with helpful citations I've missed.

My gratitude to Dr. Richard K. Bernstein is in a class by itself. I picked up his book, *Dr. Bernstein's Diabetes Solution*, on the day I was diagnosed in 1998. What I read there contradicted everything my doctors told me. But unlike what they told me, his advice worked. It was radical back then. By now it is almost mainstream. His legacy will be a generation of people with diabetes who do not develop the diabetic complications caused by tragically flawed medical advice.

Words are not enough to thank my life partner, Peter Atwood, for all that he does, including—let's be honest here—bringing home far too much artisanal chocolate.

Index

Made in the USA
Las Vegas, NV
03 September 2021

29568622R00142